To Your Health

OTHER BOOKS AUTHORED OR COAUTHORED
BY BARRY FOX, PH.D.

The Arthritis Cure
Foods to Heal By
Natural Relief for Pain and Depression
Alternative Healing
The Healthy Prostate
Beyond Positive Thinking
Making Miracles
Immune for Life
Wake Up! You're Alive
DLPA to End Chronic Pain and Depression
The Beverly Hills Medical Diet

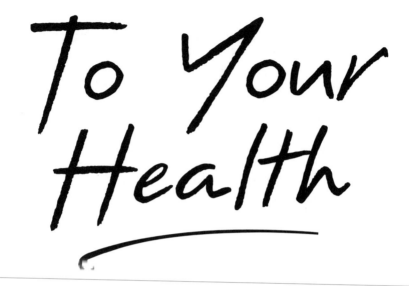

To Your Health

THE HEALING POWER OF ALCOHOL

Barry Fox, Ph.D.

St. Martin's Press
New York

Production Editor: David Stanford Burr
Design: Irving Perkins Associates

Library of Congress Cataloging-in-Publication Data

Fox, Barry.
    To your health : the healing power of alcohol /
Barry Fox.
        p.   cm.
    ISBN 0-312-15226-4
    1. Alcoholic beverages—Therapeutic use.   I. Title.
RM257.A42F68   1997
615'.7828—dc21   96-37425
                                                               CIP

First Edition: July 1997

10   9   8   7   6   5   4   3   2   1

To my wife, Nadine

Contents

Introduction by Arnold Fox, M.D.   1

ONE   Alcohol, the Unrecognized Healer   3

TWO   A Brief History of Alcohol   7

THREE   Alcohol Facts and Stats   26

FOUR   How Alcohol Protects the Heart   38

FIVE   Reducing the Risk of Stroke   49

SIX   Alcohol Fights Stress   59

SEVEN   Drinking, Good Health, and Long Life   67

EIGHT   Alcohol and the Healthy Lifestyle   80

NINE   Beware of Excess   103

TEN   Alcohol Q&A   115

APPENDIX 1   Alcohol and the Heart in the Medical Literature   125

APPENDIX 2   Alcohol and Stroke in the Medical Literature   157

Notes   161

Bibliography   171

Acknowledgments

I'D LIKE TO THANK my wife, Nadine, and my mother, Hannah, for carefully reading the manuscript hot off the computer to check for errors. Thanks to Lina Petrucco of Petrucco Wines in Butrio, Italy, for providing me with information on the history of wine and wine making, and of course, to Jeff Davidson, DTM.

Please Note

THE INFORMATION PRESENTED in the book is for educational purposes only, and is not intended to replace the advice of your physician. Should you have any health problems or questions, see your physician. Neither is the information in this book intended to suggest that you should start drinking or increase your consumption of alcohol-containing beverages.

This book was written without the monetary support of the alcohol industry or any alcohol beverage companies

Introduction

I REMEMBER THE first time I dissected a human body, way back in medical school in the 1950s. Our old anatomy professor (how old fifty seemed to me back then!) pointed to one of the cadavers we were to work on and said: "This is Mr. Jenkins. He was a heavy drinker, which means that his coronary arteries will be clear."

He was right. When we looked into the arteries supplying blood to Mr. Jenkins's heart, they were clear. Time and time again I examined the arteries of drinkers, always surprised to see that they were not nearly as clogged as those of the nondrinkers.

Well, it's only taken modern medicine forty years to catch up to what the older doctors knew back in the 1950s: alcohol has a protective effect upon the heart. It has many other benefits as well, benefits that many doctors have quietly been utilizing for years. I say "quietly" because any physician who openly prescribed small amounts of alcohol risked damaging his professional reputation.

Fortunately, mounting evidence is forcing the medical establishment to admit that alcohol can be helpful to certain people in certain cases. The medical literature is filled with studies attesting to alcohol's beneficial effects on the heart, and there are other studies showing that it also protects against ischemic stroke and ameliorates the often deleterious effects of stress. Other papers have looked at alcohol's ability to help people suffering from the physical and mental ailments related to aging, or those weighed down by certain mental illnesses.

Alcohol is certainly not a panacea but, as you'll discover while reading this book, it has an important role to play in helping to keep us healthy and happy, and possibly in even adding years to our lives. You might accuse me of being a little biased, since the author is my son, but I think this is a wonderful book, filled with facts and easy to read.

If you don't drink, don't start now. If you do, drink modestly, for heavy drinking can harm the human mind and body in numerous ways. But whether you do or do not drink, you'll be fascinated by the information in this book.

—ARNOLD FOX, M.D.

CHAPTER ONE

Alcohol, the Unrecognized Healer

AS FAR BACK as the 1960s, medical researchers were surprised when they realized that people who drank moderate amounts of a widely used beverage seemed to have an extra measure of protection against heart attacks. Not only that, these people seemed to be living longer. Back then no one knew why, but today, after three decades of large-scale study, scientists have demonstrated that drinking moderate amounts of this common substance can:

- increase HDL, the "good" cholesterol that protects against heart disease
- guard against ischemic stroke
- make the platelets in the blood less "sticky," thus reducing the risk of an unwanted blood clot that can trigger a heart attack
- moderate some of the harmful effects of stress
- protect against gallstones
- aid diabetics by helping the body to keep blood sugar under control

And there's more. Many prestigious studies, including the American Cancer Society Study, the Kaiser Permanente Study, the British Doctor's Study, and the Japanese Physician's Study have shown that drinking moderate amounts of this amazing substance can reduce one's relative risk of dying from many causes, not just heart disease, by as much as 10–30 percent!

This health-enhancing substance is not an exotic, expensive prescription medicine. On the contrary, it is readily available and remarkably inexpensive. It comes in many forms. You can buy it in most grocery stores, and it is served in numerous restaurants. It even tastes good!

What is it? Moderate amounts of alcohol.

Large amounts of alcohol are dangerous—just as too much of a drug or any other substance can be harmful. The fact that alcohol is abused by some, however, should not make us close our eyes to the many scientifically documented benefits of alcohol, especially when those benefits may help us to overcome heart disease, the number-one killer in the United States today.

Although the idea that alcohol may help to lengthen life seems startling, this beverage has long been considered a health aid. The New and Old Testaments, for example, mention the medicinal properties of alcohol nearly two hundred times. Pliny the Elder, the famous Roman physician, noted that wine "invigorates the body." Ancient, classical, and premodern writings list the many ailments for which alcohol was prescribed, including stomach distress, insomnia, melancholy, respiratory problems, fatigue, and tapeworm. As late as the 1950s, alcohol was considered to be the second-most effective remedy for heart problems. And during the past several decades, researchers have amassed an impressive body of evidence indicating that small to moderate amounts of alcohol have many beneficial effects on health. It's clear that alcohol is rapidly moving from the murky areas of folklore and home remedy into the well-documented realm of modern medical science.

Unfortunately, well-intentioned but sometimes excessive antialcohol rhetoric has blinded many people to its potential benefits. That's a shame, for reducing heart disease, moderating the effects of stress, lowering the risk of stroke and increasing longevity can be tremendous boons to society as we struggle with the rapidly mounting costs of health care. The time is ripe for a reasoned discussion of the benefits of moderate amounts of alcohol.

Interest in the heath benefits of alcohol leapt onto the national stage in late 1991, when television's *60 Minutes* reported on the "French Paradox." Despite the fact that their diets are much higher in fat than ours, and that they smoke many more cigarettes per capita than we do here in the United States, the French suffer from 40 percent fewer heart attacks—and live an average of 2½ years longer than Americans. Now, heart disease and longevity are complex issues, so it's difficult to point to any one thing the French do or do not do that protects their hearts and lengthens their lives. However, the fact that they drink large amounts of red and white wine intrigued many scientists. Could there be a link between alcohol consumption, heart health, and longer life?

The alcohol-health debate has raged here in the United States for many years. With the publication of greater and greater amounts of positive scientific proof, more and more health experts are agreeing that light to moderate consumption could indeed contribute to good health. A major breakthrough came on 2 January 1996, when the federal government performed an about-face and acknowledged, for the first time, that drinking moderate amounts of alcohol could enhance one's health. Dr. Philip Lee, the assistant secretary of Health stated that ". . . wine with meals in moderation is beneficial."[1] Donna Shalala, secretary of Health and Human Services, agreed, adding that "food is not just fuel; it is one of life's greatest pleasures."[2]

We'll take a detailed look at alcohol, the ancient and common yet controversial substance that has been both praised and damned, by:

- exploring the many benefits of drinking small to moderate amounts of alcohol. This explanation is based on an impressive body of scientifically valid studies conducted in major laboratories and universities the world over, and published in some of the most prestigious medical peer-review journals;
- examining heart disease, stroke, stress and other ailments, explaining how moderate amounts of alcohol can help to protect against these often deadly problems;
- addressing some of the misconceptions about alcohol, showing, for example, that moderate amounts of alcohol do not make one obese.

Of course, we'll candidly address the issue of alcohol abuse, explaining how to recognize the signs of abuse and what to do if you see these signs in yourself, a loved one, or a friend.

Let me be perfectly clear: I am not promoting alcohol as a wonder drug that will cure all ills. Nor am I suggesting that everyone should drink in order to avoid heart disease or other ailments. In fact, I'm quite blunt about saying that if you are not a drinker, you should *not* start drinking just to enjoy alcohol's health benefits. If you already drink, don't use alcohol's health benefits as a reason to drink more. (As I point out in Chapter 8, you can get equal health benefits through diet, exercise, and changes in lifestyle.) And of course, everyone should be aware and wary of alcohol's well-known and potentially dangerous side effects.

I ask you, however, to take a careful look at the evidence gathered by scientists from around the world. But before delving into the research, let's look briefly at the history of alcohol.

Chapter Two

A Brief History of Alcohol

No one knows who discovered alcohol—which ancient man or woman noticed that juice dripping from some discarded fruit or grain had acquired an entirely new taste and some novel effects. But even before this discovery we humans were unknowingly acquainted with alcohol. That's because there's alcohol inside our bodies and in our foods. We can't get away from it, even if we never drink a single alcoholic beverage.

Generally speaking, alcohol is a substance in which there is a carbon atom, with all four of the carbon atom's "linking sites" connected to other atoms (meaning that the carbon atom is saturated), and one of those four "linking sites" is attached to a combination of an oxygen atom and a hydrogen atom bonded together. (The oxygen and hydrogen duo is known as a hydroxyl.)

A saturated carbon atom attached to a hydroxyl—this rather broad definition of alcohol includes a great many naturally occurring substances, including vitamin A, the lactic acid that builds up in our muscles during exercise, and methanol, which is sometimes called "wood alcohol." When we speak of alcohol, however, we usually mean *ethyl alcohol*, also known as *ethanol*. That's the primary alcohol found in wine, beer, and spirits.

Early Wine Makers

We owe our enjoyment of alcoholic beverages to yeast, the same single-celled fungi that can cause skin diseases and can make bread rise. Not confined to sterile packets, it exists in the very air that surrounds us.

The varieties of yeast used to make alcoholic beverages literally eat sugar, releasing alcohol and carbon dioxide as the waste products of their feasts. This yeast-driven process of converting sugar into alcohol and carbon dioxide is called fermentation.

The Birth of Wine

MANY CIVILIZATIONS HAVE stories detailing the birth of wine. One ancient fable tells of the titanic struggle between the gods of good and evil as the world came into being. The good forces won, but many of their number were slain during the battle. Wherever the good gods fell, grapevines grew.

Here are some other explanations for the beginnings of the vine:

Armenian—According to the traditions of this southwest Asian country, Noah planted a vineyard near Erivan after the flood. It's from this vineyard that all grapes are descended.

Basque—Legend has it that grapevines were first brought to this mountainous region between France and Spain from places unknown by a man named Ano. (And *ano* is the Basque word for "wine.")

Egyptian—Osiris, god of plants and the afterlife, taught men how to make wine.

Greek—Ancient Greek legends tell us that Zeus, the ruler of the gods, sent a great flood upon the Earth to destroy all mankind, which was evil. Only one man and one woman were allowed to survive. In one version of the story, their son Orestheus planted the first grapevine. In another, their daughter Amphictyon was taught how to make wine by Dionysus, the Greek god of wine.

The great Greek poet Homer describes how wine saved the life of the hero Odysseus. While sailing home after the Trojan wars, Odysseus and his men were captured by the one-

continued

8

eyed Cyclops, who liked to eat humans. Odysseus gave the monster, who was used to weak beverages, strong wine to drink. When the Cyclops fell into a drunken sleep, Odysseus put out the monster's eye and escaped.

Islamic—According to the Koran, the first vineyard was planted by Noah's son Ham. Satan also had a hand in the planting, sprinkling peacock blood on the ground, ape blood on the leaves, lion blood on the green grapes, and swine blood on the mature grapes. Thus, thanks to the Devil, the first drink of wine animates the drinker, makes him colorful like a peacock. The second drink makes him happy, so he leaps like an ape. The third fills him with fury and fight, like a lion, while the fourth turns him into a swine, groveling on the ground and passing out.

Jewish—Although the Old Testament does not say who actually discovered wine, it does tell how, immediately after the great flood, Noah planted a vineyard and drank of the wine (and got so drunk that he passed out, naked, in his tent!).

Persian—During the reign of an ancient, semimythical king named Jamsheed, grapes were stored in jars. The grapes in one jar began to foam and smell bad, so they were believed to be poisonous and were set aside. A despondent member of Jamsheed's harem decided to kill herself by drinking the poison. Instead of dying, however, she felt much better. When she told the king what had happened, he ordered that wine be made for the entire court to drink.

The first wine maker may have been a cavewoman who forgot about some honey she had stored away, returning weeks later to find that it had changed. She didn't know about fermentation, about the airborne yeast that had wafted onto her honey and converted its sugar into alcohol and carbon dioxide. But she—or someone else—probably quickly realized that the odd-tasting "aged honey" had some appealing qualities. Or perhaps the first alcoholic drink sampled by early man was a tiny pool of fluid that had seeped from a piece of rotting fruit that had been set upon by yeast.

Either fruits or honey are believed to be the first sources of alcoholic beverages because they contain simple sugars, such as fructose, which yeast can digest. The barley, rye, corn, and similar grains used to make beer, whiskey, and other alcoholic beverages have more complex sugars in the form of starches. Before yeast can make alcohol from grains, their complex starches must be broken down into the simple sugars that yeast can ingest.

At various unrecorded times, civilizations all over the world learned how to carefully "rot" certain foods in order to produce alcohol. They didn't know exactly what was happening, what caused fermentation or how it worked, but they gradually learned to control the process. Grapes, honey, apples, peaches, dates, rice, barley, millet, milk, and even the sap from palm trees were used as raw materials for the mysterious process that somehow produced alcohol. The grape eventually became the favored fruit for making wine because it could be grown in many climates, it matured quickly and it fermented smoothly. And compared to fruit trees, grapevines produced relatively large crops.

The remnants of grapes have been uncovered in Turkish, Syrian, Jordanian, and Lebanese cities dating back as far as 8000 B.C., but no one knows exactly when man began to cultivate grapes for wine, rather than simply picking those that happened to grow nearby. Archeologists tell us that perhaps as early as 5000 B.C. the Egyptians cultivated and fermented grapes of the *Vitis sylvestris* species. And by about 4000 B.C. *Vitis vinifera*, the best wine-producing species of grape, was being cultivated in the Near East. (*Vinifera* means "bearer of wine.") The earliest written records relating to wine are inscriptions on the seals of wine vessels found in the tombs of the pharaohs. Archeologists have also uncovered the remains of a large-scale winery, dating back to 600 B.C., near Jerusalem.

THE SPREAD OF THE VINE

When Homer wrote his *Iliad* and *Odyssey* in the eighth century B.C., wine was already a staple drink in Greece. In fact, a typical breakfast for an ancient Greek included bread dipped in wine, and the Greek word for eating breakfast meant "to drink undiluted wine." And drink wine the Greeks did, flavoring it with spices, herbs, honey, vegetables, raisins, and more, or using it as a medicine for many ailments. Greek traders brought their favorite wine to colonies in Asia Minor, Italy, and Spain, planting *Vitis vinifera* vines whenever and wherever possible.

Grape growing was well established in Italy by about 200 B.C. When the Roman Empire began spreading from the Italian peninsula up to England, Germany, France, and other parts of Europe, its armies and merchants took with them their preferred wines, vines, and production methods. During the several hundred years that Rome ruled the known world, vineyards were established in the Danube, Rhine, Burgundy, Bordeaux, and other regions of Europe that later came be to known for fine wines.

Vine cultivation suffered when the Roman Empire weakened and finally collapsed in the fourth and fifth centuries A.D. During the Middle Ages that followed, wine and wine making were handled primarily by the monasteries, whose monks were learned men who had the time to labor in the fields. These monasteries were often given grants of land or existing vineyards to cultivate. In fact, the Church was the primary producer of wine for much of this dark period. Some Christian orders took a great deal of pride in the wine they manufactured, going to great lengths to ensure quality. Legend has it that the Cistercian monks of Cîteaux literally tasted the soil to make sure that it would produce good grapes before planting their vines.

A Benedictine monk named Dom Perignon is credited with some great advances in wine making. As cellar master of an abbey in France's Champagne region in the late seventeenth and early eighteenth centuries, he pioneered the blending of wines to improve flavor and other qualities. He also solved the problem of *vin diable* ("devil wine"), also known as "cork popper." Grapes were fermented to make wine, but certain wines refermented themselves in the spring. If these wines had been stored in closed containers, they were liable to explode as carbon dioxide levels built. Dom Perignon solved the problem by having the wine poured into thick bottles covered with strong stoppers that were tied securely to the bottles.

Disaster struck the French wine industry in the mid-1800s when much of the wine exported by French vintners turned sour or vinegary. The good name of France was at stake, declared Emperor Louis-Napoleon, and something must be done immediately! The famed scientist Louis Pasteur was called upon to solve the problem. After studying many wine samples, Pasteur realized that the problem was caused by certain bacteria in wines. His solution was simple: seal wine in airtight bottles, then heat it. This process, called pasteurization, killed the existing bacteria in the wine and prevented new bacteria from contaminating the fluid.

But no sooner had that problem been solved when a new, greater

11

crisis enveloped French vineyards and threatened to destroy the entire European wine industry. It seems that native American grapevines brought to Europe had carried with them a parasite called *Phylloxera vastatrix* ("the devastator"). American vines were immune to the tiny pest, but European vines withered when their roots were attacked by phylloxera. Many vineyards were saved when European vines were grafted onto the sturdy American roots. So that fine French wine you drink today may have been made from a mixture of American and French vines!

WINE AND MEDICINE

No one knows when wine's medicinal uses were discovered, or when wine was first used to cleanse wounds or make water safe to drink. Ancient Egyptians and other peoples used wine to treat respiratory and urinary problems, upset stomachs, constipation, and tapeworms. Hundreds of years before the advent of the Common Era, the Jewish Talmud noted that "Where wine is lacking, drugs become necessary." Medical texts written in India during the same time period praise wine for its ability to invigorate the mind and body while relieving fatigue, sorrow, and insomnia. Hippocrates of Greece, the father of medicine, used wine to treat fever, to help the body dispose of excess fluid, to dull pain, and to improve general health. But he insisted that wine should be imbibed either warm or cool, never hot or cold. Drinking too much hot wine, he warned, could turn one into an idiot, while cold wine would cause fever, chills, and convulsions. Christian texts written hundreds of years later agreed that wine could be a useful medicine. St. Paul suggested using "a little wine for thine stomach's sake and thine often infirmities."

Although wine had been used medicinally for perhaps thousands of years, it's likely that alcohol itself was not isolated until approximately 1100 A.D. by doctors at the medical school in Salerno, Italy. Through the process of distillation, alcohol was separated from wine and recognized as the active medicinal ingredient.[1] Doctors and others in this period could hardly restrain themselves in their praise of this new medicinal fluid, which they named *aqua vitae* ("the water of life"). One went so far as to claim that it was "an emanation of the divinity, an element newly revealed to men but hid from antiquity, because the human race was then too young to need this beverage destined to revive the energies of modern decrepitude."[2] Considered a powerful

Three Strikes and You're Out

EARLY EXPERTS RECOGNIZED the health benefits of wine, but cautioned against excess. In about 375 B.C., the Greek writer Eubulus explained the situation thusly: "Three bowls do I mix for the temperate: one to health, which they empty first, the second to love and pleasure, the third to sleep. When this bowl is drunk up, wise guests go home. The fourth bowl is ours no longer, but belongs to violence; the fifth to uproar, the sixth to drunken revelry, the seventh to black eyes, the eighth is the policeman's, the ninth belongs to biliousness, and the tenth to madness and hurling the furniture."[3]

medicine, it was made in and dispensed by monasteries and apothecaries. During the next several hundred years, the medicine called *aqua vitae* gradually evolved into a fluid that one drank for pleasure, and the process of distillation was used to make a variety of alcoholic beverages, including gin and whiskey.

Until relatively recent times, alcohol was used by doctors to cleanse wounds and help patients endure the pain of surgery. As late as the 1950s, doctors prescribed moderate amounts of alcohol for a variety of ailments, including trouble with the heart, anxiety, stress, and problems with conception.

WINE AND RELIGION

After escaping from Egypt, crossing the Red Sea, and wandering for forty years in the desert, the Israelites came to the Promised Land. Moses sent men to spy on the land. The Old Testament tells us that the spies "came unto the brook of Eschol, and cut down from thence a branch with one cluster of grapes, and they bore it between them upon a staff." The grapes were proof that the land was fruitful and good.

Wine has always played an important role in Jewish religion and

Beware the "False Cure"

THERE'S NOTHING LIKE a shot of whiskey to warm you on a cold night, right? Wrong. Alcohol does *not* warm the body. It fools us into thinking that it does so by opening the small blood vessels close to the surface of the skin. With warm blood rushing from the body's vital organs toward the skin we feel a temporary flush, but all we've done is transfer warmth from one part of the body to another. If you're cold, a sweater or blanket is much better than a drink. And don't give someone else a drink to "warm up"—you might end up doing just the opposite.

culture. In ancient times, mourners were offered ten cups of wine at the funerals of their loved ones. To this day, Jews the world over welcome the Sabbath by blessing, then drinking, wine. Every year at the Passover celebration, four cups of wine are enjoyed. Two cups of wine are used in Jewish weddings, and one at the ritual circumcisions of newborn boys. Despite this abundance of wine in Jewish culture, however, alcoholism is severely frowned upon and Jews are traditionally a sober people. The rabbis and sages of Judaism have insisted that wine should be used to enhance reasoning and joy, never for intoxication. They point to Psalm 104, which notes that "Wine maketh glad the heart of man," then to Proverbs 20:1, which reminds us that "Wine is a mocker, strong drink is raging."

Wine has also long been intertwined with Christian beliefs and practices. The first miracle Jesus performed was to convert water into wine at a wedding. At the Last Supper, Jesus had his followers sip from a cup of wine, instructing them to "Drink ye all of it, for this is my blood of the new testament which is shed for many for the remission of sins. But I say to you, I will not drink henceforth of this fruit of the vine until that day when I drink it new with you in my Father's kingdom."[4]

And so, sacred Communion is not complete without wine, as St. Thomas Aquinas explains: "The Sacrament of the Eucharist can only be performed with wine from the vine, for it is the will of Christ Jesus, who chose wine when He ordained this sacrament . . ."[5]

The third great Western religion, Islam, forbade the drinking of alcohol. The Koran states that "Satan seeks to stir up enmity and hatred among you by means of wine and gambling, and to keep you from the remembrance of Allah and from your prayers. Will you not abstain from them?" The penalty for imbibing during the life of the Prophet Mohammed was forty lashes, increased to eighty by his successor, the Caliph Umar.

Within the hundred years following of the death of the Prophet Mohammed in the seventh century A.D., alcohol had been officially banished from Arabia, Palestine, Egypt, and other parts of North Africa, Mesopotamia, Spain, Portugal, Crete, and other lands conquered by the energetic Muslims. However, the faithful are promised that when they die, they shall ascend to Paradise, where they will "drink of a pure wine, securely sealed, whose very dregs are musk; . . . a wine tempered with the water of Tasnim . . ."[6]

The prohibition against alcohol deprived Arab physicians of one of their best medicines. It did not, however, stop many wealthy and powerful Arab rulers from drinking. They justified imbibing by arguing over exactly what constituted a wine, by claiming that wine made from dates did not count, by asserting that it was only drunkenness (not drinking) that was prohibited, and by otherwise bending the rules.

BEER FOR THE COMMON FOLK

As is the case with wine, the origins of beer are shrouded in the mysteries of ancient times. Egyptian legends tell us that Osiris, the god of life and agriculture, taught his people how to brew beer thousands of years before Christ was born. Writing in the early third century B.C., the Greek Athenaeus offered a different explanation, stating that beer was invented in Egypt so that the poorer folk who could not afford wine would have a beverage of their own. Other early authors argue that beer was known before wine, so we may never know the true origins of the "common folks drink." But we do know that beer was a popular drink in ancient times. As early as 1750 B.C., the Code of Hammurabi made it illegal for Babylonian beer sellers to adulterate their beer, or otherwise defraud customers. (Barmaids who cheated their customers were to be tossed into the river as punishment!)

Beer has been made from barley, millet, corn, rice, and almost every other grain. But airborne yeast falling on grains can't immediately turn the sugars in grain into alcohol, the way it does with the sugars in fruit

The Beer Facts

The ones who love beer the most—The people of the Czech Republic consume the most beer: 295.9 pints per person in 1993.[7]

Oldest beer—May have been in the remains of a jug dating back to roughly 3500 B.C., found at Godin Tepe, Iran.[8]

Oldest brewer—Germany's Weihenstepha Brewery dates back to A.D. 1040.[9]

First beer brewed in the United States—Sir Walter Raleigh of Roanoke Colony, in what is now Virginia, brewed the first batch of beer in 1587 in what became the United States.[10]

First beer manufactured in the United States—The first brewer/manufacturer was John Wagner of Philadelphia, who began manufacturing beer in 1840.[11]

First canned beer sold in the United States—On 24 January, 1935, the Krueger Brewing Company offered the first canned beer to retail customers.[12]

Strongest beer in the world—The Parish Brewery in Somerby, England, brews Baz's Super Brew, which is 23 percent alcohol by volume.[13]

Strongest beer in the United States—The Boston Beer Company brews Samuel Adams Triple Bock which, by volume, is 17.7 percent alcohol.[14]

Largest brewer in the world—Anheuser-Busch, Inc., owns thirteen breweries in the United States. The company's Budweiser is the world's best-selling beer.[15]

or honey. That's because grain sugars are bound up in the form of complex starches, which yeast can't digest. So beer brewing begins with the soaking of the grains in water. In essence, the grains are allowed to sprout (like the beans or seeds that become "sprouts" for salads and sandwiches). During the sprouting process, enzymes in the grains "nibble" on the starches, chopping them up into the simple sugars that yeast can then convert into alcohol.

Sprouting is an ancient procedure for making grains and beans soft and edible. So perhaps beer was "invented" when someone forgot to eat a bowl of sprouted grain and it was fermented by airborne yeast. But sprouting is not the only way to convert the starches in grains into simple sugars. The native inhabitants of Peru had a unique method of making beer: Women cooked grains until they were palatable, chewed them, then spat them out. Their saliva digested (broke up) the starches in the grains, turning them into sugars that yeast could consume. The grains were then boiled, cooled, and filtered to make beer. Yet another technique, native to Asia, uses a starch-splitting mold called *koji*, which grows on rice. Koji is used to make sake, which, because it comes from rice, is a beer and not a wine.

Beer, which the Romans thought was a barbarian drink, naturally spread through Europe after the barbarians captured Rome. (Wine was still available, but was more expensive.) During the Middle Ages, hops were added to beer to enhance the flavor and prevent spoilage. The British, who called their beer "ale," did not like hops, most likely because early hopped beers happened to be rather light. So far did the British turn their noses up at hops that in 1484 the City of London made it a crime to add hops to ale! Other cities took similar steps to distinguish between beer (which had hops) and ale (which didn't). The unhopped ale versus hopped beer battle continued, with separate guilds for makers of ale and beer being formed. But by the late 1600s the hop lovers had won. From then on, hops were added to both ale and beer.

Early beer (and ale) was stored in large, open tanks. This means that it was "flat," since the carbon dioxide produced by the yeast (which makes beer bubbly) would have risen to the top and dissipated. But when beer began to be stored in corked bottles, the carbon dioxide did not escape and bubbly beer came into being. According to an old story, it was the dean of St. Paul's Cathedral in London who first stumbled across bubbly beer. Sometime in the late 1500s, the dean took a bottle of corked beer with him on a fishing trip. He forgot about the bottle for a few days and when he finally retrieved and opened it, was startled to see the cork fly off the bottle with a loud "pop." Flat beer remained the rule, however, for hundreds of years until closed airtight kegs were developed and carbonation could be controlled.

Brewing Beer

MODERN BEER, WHICH is made primarily from barley, is brewed in several steps:

Germination: The barley is placed in water and allowed to sprout (germinate). Enzymes in the barley break down the grain's starches, cell walls, and protein.

Malting—The sprouting barley is placed in temperature-controlled revolving drums to encourage the production of the starch-splitting enzymes. Malting also prevents the growing barley sprouts from using too much of their energy supplies to grow the long "tails" characteristic of sprouted grains and beans.

Kilning—The malted barley is heated and dried to halt the sprouting and temporarily deactivate the starch-splitting enzymes. The higher the temperature used during kilning, the more colorful and flavorful the beer will be.

Mashing—The ground-up barley kernels (the *malt*) are soaked in hot water for several hours. The minerals in the water become part of the beer, so the brewer carefully selects and/or alters the water used. (For example, calcium in the water makes for a better tasting beer than does magnesium or sodium.)

Further flavoring—Sugar, rice flakes, ground-up corn, or other substances may be added, along with either hops or hop extracts. Hops, which are female flowers of a vine called the *Humulus lupulus*, add flavor and aroma to the beer.

Fermentation—Now that the barley grains have been converted into a sweet liquid, yeast is added to convert the barley's sugar into alcohol and carbon dioxide.

Conditioning—The beer is treated to remove odors, add carbonation, skim out undesirable particles, et cetera. Preservatives, antigushing agents, and other additives may be introduced into the fluid. Some beers are *lagered,* which means that they are placed in cold storage to improve the taste.

Where the Words Come From

Alcohol—from the Arabic *al kohl*, which was a fine powder used as eye shadow.

Al kohl later came to mean the essence of any substance, and was used by a German alchemist of the 1500s to describe the essence of wine.

Beer—from the Roman word *biber*, which means "drink."

Brandy—derived from the German words *brannten wein* or *Bernewyn*, which mean "burnt wine."

Champagne—a sparkling wine named for its birthplace, the Champagne region of France.

Cordial—this term for after-dinner drinks comes from the Latin *cor*, which means "heart." (Once it had been identified and isolated, alcohol was felt to be a medicine for the heart and other parts of the body.)

Gin—from *jenever*, the Dutch word for the juniper that was used to flavor the drink.

Liquor—originally meaning simply "liquid," it is a popular term for alcoholic spirits.

Intoxication—from the Greek *toxikon*, which means a poison used for arrows.

Port—the name originally given to any wine that came from Portugal.

Sherry—a corruption of "Jerez de la Frontera," the Spanish town where sherry is made.

Vodka—derived from the Russian word for "water."

Whiskey—comes from *uisge beatha*, which is Gaelic for *aqua vitae* (the "water of life"). In England and Canada, whiskey is spelled "whisky."

DISTILLED SPIRITS

To distill means "to let fall drop by drop." And so the ancients boiled their wine or beer until the alcohol and other aromatic elements turned to steam and rose up out of the bubbling vat. The steam was then captured and allowed to fall, drop by drop, into a different vessel. This vessel contained a new alcoholic beverage—distilled spirits or liquor—which was much stronger than the original and had a different taste and other qualities.

Distilling works because the alcohol and other important elements in the beverage have lower boiling points than does water. This means that they will turn to steam and rise from the original fluid before the water does. What rises, therefore, has a greater concentration of alcohol than the original wine or beer, along with a new taste and aroma. The alcohol in the new fluid is, of course, unchanged. The difference is simply that there is more of it for a given volume of liquid.

It is not known who first realized that a mild wine could be made into a strong distilled spirit. The Chinese were certainly among the initial distillers, mastering the process as early as 800 B.C. Through repeated distillations, they turned rice beer (made up of about 10 percent alcohol) into a strong drink called arrack, which contained some 40 percent alcohol.

Distilling was undoubtedly discovered and rediscovered at various times and places throughout history, despite the credit given to the doctors at the medical school in Salerno, Italy. The public was not nearly as enthusiastic as the doctors about this awful-tasting concoction, which they often called *aqua ardens,* or "fire water." But the learned doctors were determined to cure their patients with their *aqua vitae.* So they flavored their medicine with a spoonful of sugar or anything else that would help it go down. Little by little the unpalatable medicine became a strong but tasty drink with all the beneficial effects of wine and more, because the distilled spirits were much stronger than the wine from which they came. Their appetite for these powerful alcoholic beverages whetted, people around the globe experimented with new concoctions, giving birth to gin, whiskey, rum, vodka, and numerous other distilled spirits. Although *aqua vitae* continued to be used as a medicine, it was even more widely used as the base for pleasurable drinks.

Let's take a brief look at some of the more popular distilled spirits or liquors:

Why Distill?

WHY GO THROUGH the distillation process in order to produce strong drinks? Why not simply produce wine or beer with a higher alcohol content?

The fermentation of fruits and grains is naturally self-limiting because alcohol is, by nature, a poison. When the alcohol content of a food being fermented rises to about 15 percent, the alcohol kills off the very yeast that created it. No matter how sweet the fruit or grain is, no matter how much sugar it has for the yeast to eat, the alcohol content cannot rise much above 15 percent. The only way to increase a drink's alcohol content is through distillation.

Bourbon—Born in Kentucky, bourbon is a uniquely American form of whiskey. So says the U.S. Congress, which in 1964 proclaimed bourbon to be a "distinctive product of the United States." The Reverend Elija Craig is credited with devising the recipe for bourbon, which is distilled from a mix of corn, barley, wheat, and other grains. The reverend's drink was dubbed "bourbon" because he happened to have his still in Bourbon County. Today, federal regulations require that bourbon be made from a whiskey mash consisting of at least 51 percent corn, wheat, rye, malted barley, or malted grain. It must be aged in charred oak barrels and be at least 80 proof.

Brandy—Legend has it that a Dutch sea captain carrying a cargo of wine wanted to save space, so he heated his wine to "burn off" the water, intending to add it back when he arrived in port. But when he tasted the fluid he distilled from the wine, he decided to leave it as is. Originally know as *brannten wein* or *Bernewyn,* which means "burnt wine," brandy is made from grapes, apples, and other fruits.

Cognac—Cognac is a type of brandy made from grapes grown in the Cognac region of France.

Gin—Although the English often take a bow for inventing gin, most scholars give the credit to a seventeenth-century chemist from Holland named Franciscus de la Boe. La Boe was mixing juniper berry oil with pure alcohol in an attempt to create a new, inexpensive medicine that would, among other things, flush excess fluid out of the body. The juniper-flavored alcohol did not pass muster as a medicine, but it quickly became a popular drink in England. The timing was fortuitous; gin became available just as the British were looking for an alternative to heavily taxed, expensive French wines. Today, Dutch gin is made from barley, corn, rye, and juniper berries, while English gin is a mix of corn and barley, with lemon, orange, coriander, licorice, and other flavorings added.

Port—The name of the wine comes from its country of origin, Portugal. Although the English originally called just about any wine coming from Portugal "port," the word is now applied to a sweet, fortified wine made from red grapes, mixed with brandy. Traditional methods call for the grapes to be walked on by human feet for twelve hours and for the wine to be aged in barrels for up to fifty years.

Rum—We may have Christopher Columbus to thank for rum. It's believed that he brought sugarcane to the West Indies, where it was distilled into rum. Rum quickly became popular in the New World: Shortly before the Revolution the average colonist was enjoying an average of four gallons per year. And rum played an important role in the American Revolution, for the colonists were just as upset at the taxes that England levied on rum as they were at the tea tax. (Had a different ship been in the harbor that celebrated night, the Boston Tea Party might have been the Boston Rum Party instead!) And legend has it that Paul Revere cooled off with a glass of rum after his midnight ride. (Another version of the story claims that Mr. Revere began his ride in silence, only shouting, "The British are coming!" after stopping for a quick but hefty dose of rum along the way!)

Scotch—A form of whiskey thought by some to be the original distilled spirit, scotch is intimately linked to Scotland, the land of its birth, where over 3,500 brands are manufactured today. Once drunk "single," it did not become popular outside of Scotland until the mid-1800s when merchants began mixing together scotch whiskeys from different distilleries to create milder-tasting blended scotch. Most Scotch whiskey is distilled in one of four areas of Scotland; the Highlands, which produces a light, full-bodied, and fragrant malt; the Lowlands, from whence comes a light and soft liquid; Islay, which makes a thick and peaty drink; and Campbeltown, where the scotch is made rich and full bodied. Scotch was responsible for a colorful addition to the language back in the 1920s, during Prohibition. A smuggler named Captain McCoy guaranteed that his scotch was the real thing, giving us our expression "the real McCoy."

Sherry—Sherry is a fortified wine born in the Spanish town of Jerez de la Frontera, which the English mistakenly pronounced "sherry." Sherry was first noticed by the Western world when the Romans defeated the Carthaginians and claimed southern Spain as a prize of war. The Romans thought that sherry was the only Spanish wine worthy of praise, and it has been quite popular in England since the late 1500s.

Tequila—Like mescal and pulque, tequila is made from the juice of the *blue agave*, a tall, cactuslike plant that grows in the desert. (We who live north of the border call the agave the "century plant.") It's believed that tequila (named for the town of Tequila, Mexico) can be traced back to a milky, alcoholic beverage that the Aztecs made from the agave. Today there are three types of tequila: the 80-proof silver tequila, the gold tequila which has been aged for up to four years in oak vats, and the *anejo* tequila made from 100 percent blue agave. By Mexican law, a bottle cannot be labeled "tequila" unless it contains at least 51 percent blue agave and was made in Tequila or certain designated regions of the country.

Vodka—This strong alcoholic beverage made from grains originated in Russia, Poland, and adjacent lands. It was traditionally brewed with a high alcohol content, and with little taste or aroma from other compounds, but flavored vodkas have become more popular in recent years. Little-known in the United States until the late 1940s, vodka now accounts for some 25 percent of the distilled spirits market.

Whiskey—Both the Irish and the Scots claim to have invented whiskey, which is bottled at a minimum 80 proof. Scotch-Irish immigrants settling in Pennsylvania brought their whiskey with them and, shortly after the Revolution, whiskey replaced rum as the favored drink in the newborn nation. Although it can be made from many different grains, American whiskey is usually distilled from corn and rye, with lesser amounts of barley, millet, and sorghum.

A POTPOURRI OF FACTS

What Constitutes One Drink?

Most sources define a drink as 10–12 grams of ethyl alcohol, which is the amount found in 12 ounces of regular beer *or* 5 ounces of wine *or* 1½ ounces of 80-proof distilled spirits.

Are All Alcoholic Drinks Equal?

Alcohol is alcohol, whether in beer, wine, or distilled spirits. There is an *equivalence* between standard drinks, with each containing approximately the same amount of alcohol. Whether you drink a standard glass of wine containing 5 ounces of fluid, a 12-ounce can of beer or a 1¼–1½-ounce shot of whiskey, you're getting the same amount of alcohol (about 10 grams, or ½ ounce).

How Many Calories Are in a Drink?

The number of calories per drink varies from brand to brand. Use these figures, provided by the federal government, as a general guide:

12 ounces of regular beer—150 calories
5 ounces of wine—100 calories
1½ ounces of 80-proof distilled spirits—100 calories

What Does "Proof" Mean?

A beverage's proof is twice the percent of alcohol in the drink. (Actually, the proof is slightly higher than that in the United States, but doubling the alcohol content is close enough.) Thus, a beverage containing 5 percent alcohol is 10 proof, while one composed of 40 percent alcohol is 80 proof.

Hundreds of years ago, buyers checked the potency of an alcoholic beverage by heating a sample to evaporate the alcohol (which burns off at a lower temperature than water). The beverage was considered to be good if at least slightly more than half of the fluid burned off.

Why Is One Type of Grape Better than Another for Making Wine?

There are many factors, some of which are entirely subjective. However, an important characteristic of wine grapes is their sugar and acid contents. Good wine grapes need plenty of sugar to be converted into alcohol, and enough natural acid to prevent the growth of unwanted bacteria and other microbes.

Why Are Wine Bottles Stored Lying Down?

Wine bottles are laid on their sides so that the wine will remain in contact with the cork and keep it moist. If the cork dries out, it may shrink and allow oxygen to come in contact with the wine, thereby spoiling it.

Sweet Wine versus Table Wine

In general, table wines are "dry" because most of the sugar in the grapes from which they come has been fermented by yeast. But when sweet wines (also known as dessert wines) are made, the fermentation process is controlled to ensure that enough sugar remains in the wine to give it a sweet taste.

Why Are Some Alcoholic Beverages Aged in Wood Kegs?

Wood kegs allow oxygen to seep in, improving the taste or other qualities of the beverage through oxidation. The wood may also flavor and/or color the fluid.

Wine and Science

Many of science's great minds have studied fermentation, including Louis Pasteur, who was the first to analyze and describe the process. The field of microbiology was created by scientists studying fermentation and alcohol in the nineteenth century. Our word "enzyme" comes from the Greek word for "in yeast," since yeast was the first material discovered that contained tiny "spark plugs" capable of transforming one substance into another.

CHAPTER THREE

Alcohol Facts and Stats

ETHYL ALCOHOL, THE primary alcohol found in alcoholic beverages, is a clear and colorless liquid with a relatively simple chemical structure. But behind the apparent simplicity is a complex substance with myriad and seemingly contradictory affects on the mind and body.

Although it comes "packaged" as hundreds of different types of drinks, once inside the body all ethyl alcohol behaves the same way, regardless of the source. It doesn't matter whether it came from beer, wine, or hard liquor, from vintage champagne or the keg at a fraternity party—all ethyl alcohol has the same effect on the body. After passing through the mouth and traveling down the esophagus, the fluid passes from the stomach and intestines directly into the bloodstream, where it immediately begins to affect the nervous system and other parts of the body. (There is some evidence suggesting that very small amounts of alcohol may be metabolized or "deactivated" in the stomach, and hence never make it into the bloodstream.[1] Most alcohol, however, enters the bloodstream without much delay.

How rapidly alcohol is absorbed into the bloodstream depends on several factors, including:

- how much is consumed in a given amount of time
- body size
- sex
- metabolism
- the amount and type of food and fluid already in the stomach

Time—Once in the bloodstream, alcohol passes easily into the brain and other parts of the body. Ninety percent or more is eventually metabolized by the liver, with the rest passing out of the body through respiration, perspiration, and urination. The concentration of alcohol in the blood peaks between sixty and ninety minutes after drinking, then begins to taper off as it is converted by the liver into carbon dioxide and water. But the liver can only process eight to nine grams of alcohol per hour. If you drink slowly, perhaps sipping a glass of wine during dinner or nursing a drink throughout the evening, your liver will be able to keep your blood alcohol level relatively low. But if you down the same amount of alcohol all at once, it will circulate through your body for some time before the liver can deal with it all.

Size—Larger people can usually handle more alcohol because they have more blood and body fluids to dilute it.

Sex—Women tend to be affected by alcohol faster, longer, and more intensely than men, largely because they weigh less and have a higher percentage of body fat. This translates to lowered amounts of bodily fluids to dilute the alcohol. Research suggests that women also produce fewer "alcohol busting" enzymes than do men, and may be more susceptible to the effects of alcohol at specific points in their monthly cycles.

Metabolism—The rate at which alcohol is metabolized varies from individual to individual. Some people metabolize a little faster, while others are a bit slower.

Food and fluid already in the stomach—Before alcohol can have any effect on the body (other than to possibly irritate the lining of the gastrointestinal tract), it must pass from the stomach and intestines into the bloodstream. The passage is slowed if there is already food in the stomach, for the alcohol will have to wait its turn to be absorbed. That's why eating before or in conjunction with drinking helps to slow the uptake of alcohol into the bloodstream. Fatty foods are especially helpful, as they stay in the digestive tract the longest. West Africans used to rely on peanuts, while American Indians ate raw almonds to keep from becoming drunk.

How Much Alcohol Is in Beer, Wine, and Spirits?

THE AMOUNT VARIES from drink to drink and even brand to brand, but in general:

• Most beer is 4.5–5.5 percent alcohol, with some "light" beers having less and malt beverages containing more.
• Most table wines are 10–12 percent alcohol, while fortified wines may contain 14 percent or more.
• Many spirits are about 35–37.5 percent alcohol; stronger versions of some brands contain about 40 percent, and only a few contain as much as 50 percent.

Although beer, wine, and spirits contain different amounts of alcohol, they are equivalent in that a standard 5-ounce glass of wine, a 12-ounce can of beer, and a typical 1¼–1½-ounce serving of spirits all contain the same amount of alcohol (about 10 grams, or ½ ounce).

ALCOHOL'S EFFECTS ON THE BODY

Sooner or later, the alcohol one drinks will find its way into the bloodstream, brain, and the rest of the body. Whether taken in the form of champagne, beer, tequila, or sacramental wine, alcohol acts as a local anesthetic, an irritant, and a sedative with myriad effects on the body. In relatively small amounts, alcohol can:

• make one feel lightheaded by interfering with the brain's ability to use oxygen for fuel
• produce sensations of dizziness
• depress the central nervous system
• lower inhibitions and alter behavior

- produce mood changes
- increase the heart rate
- dilate the blood vessels in the skin, making the skin look red and flushed as more blood rises to the body's surface
- increase sweating
- interfere with the brain's ability to control body temperature
- irritate the lining of the stomach
- increase urination by decreasing the levels of the antidiuretic hormones, which instruct the kidney to hold on to fluid. (And since alcohol is usually mixed with a large amount of fluid, there's even a greater need to go to the bathroom)

Relatively small amounts of alcohol can also wreak havoc on one's sex life. It lowers inhibitions, encouraging one to engage in activities that might ordinarily be avoided (such as unprotected sex). And as Shakespeare noted, drinking can be a risky proposition for men, for it "provokes the desire, but takes away the performance."[2]

THE BLOOD ALCOHOL LEVEL

How much alcohol can one safely drink without running the risk of potentially serious "side effects?" The safety level varies from individual to individual, but most people can use the blood alcohol charts as guidelines. Known as "BACs" for short, using a chart is a convenient way to estimate how much alcohol there is in a given amount of blood. We measure the grams of alcohol found in 100 milliliters of blood, calling the result "grams per deciliter," "g/dl," "grams percent," or simply "g%."

At a BAC of 0.02–0.08 g/dl, the typical person may:

- experience mood changes
- act differently and inappropriately
- have difficulty interpreting what is seen and heard
- suffer from impaired coordination
- have a diminished response to pain

At a BAC of 0.100–0.199 g/dl, there may be:

- lack of coordination
- inability to correctly interpret what is happening

Different Types of Alcohol

Ethyl alcohol—the primary alcohol found in alcoholic beverages. Also known as ethanol.

Methyl alcohol—a colorless liquid with a strong odor used as a cleaner and solvent.

Isopropyl alcohol—also known as rubbing alcohol, used by doctors to cleanse wounds. It is a poisonous solvent.

Denatured alcohol—ethyl alcohol that has been deliberately "poisoned" by being mixed with methyl alcohol, benzene, and other substances that make it smell bad and taste worse. Used to make antifreeze and other products, denatured alcohol is deliberately adulterated so people won't drink it.

- poor judgment
- slowed reaction time
- difficulty in walking and standing steadily

At a BAC of 0.200–0.299 g/dl, the drinker may suffer from:

- nausea
- vomiting

When the BAC reaches 0.300–0.399 g/dl, one is seriously intoxicated. Body temperature is lowered and partial amnesia ("blackout") is likely. People who can drink enough to push their BACs to 0.300 or more are considered alcoholics, by definition.

The damage to mind and body mounts as the BAC rises. A BAC of 0.400 g/dl can cause alcohol poisoning, coma, and death. In fact, it's estimated that half of those who manage to drink enough to push their BACs up to 0.400 will die of alcohol poisoning.

Estimating Your Blood Alcohol Level

You can use these two charts to get a quick estimate of what your BAC will be after a few drinks. The first chart is for men, the second for women. Begin by finding your weight, in pounds, along the left hand column. (It's better to be cautious, so if you're in between figures, use the lesser number.) Then move your finger to the right until you find the column for your BAC at a particular number of drinks.

MEN					
	1 drink	2 drinks	3 drinks	4 drinks	5 drinks
100 lbs.	.043	.087	.130	.174	.217
125 lbs.	.034	.069	.103	.139	.173
150 lbs.	.029	.058	.087	.116	.145
175 lbs.	.025	.050	.075	.100	.125
200 lbs	.022	.043	.065	.087	.108
225 lbs.	.019	.039	.060	.078	.097
250 lbs.	.017	.035	.052	.070	.087

WOMEN					
	1 drink	2 drinks	3 drinks	4 drinks	5 drinks
100 lbs.	.050	.101	.152	.203	.253
125 lbs.	.040	.080	.120	.162	.202
150 lbs.	.034	.068	.101	.135	.169
175 lbs.	.029	.058	.087	.117	.146
200 lbs.	.026	.050	.076	.101	.126
225 lbs.	.022	.045	.068	.091	.113
250 lbs.	.020	.041	.061	.082	.101

Of course, the blood alcohol level is not static. Once you've stopped drinking, it drops with time as the liver metabolizes the alcohol. Therefore, when:

- 1 hour has passed since your last drink, subtract 0.015 from your BAC
- 2 hours have passed since your last drink, subtract .030

- 3 hours have passed since your last drink, subtract 0.045
- 4 hours have passed since your last drink, subtract 0.060
- 5 hours have passed since your last drink, subtract 0.075
- 6 hours have passed since your last drink, subtract 0.090

Please remember: These charts are only guidelines. Your reaction to alcohol may differ. When figuring your BAC, always err on the side of caution.

THE SET AND SETTING

Although alcohol's effects on the human body are well defined and unavoidable, they can be modified. We can control or significantly influence several factors that play a large role in determining how we respond to alcohol, including how it is consumed, where it is consumed, why it is consumed, with whom we are drinking, and our expectations concerning alcohol.

Where and why it is consumed, with whom we share a drink, and our expectations are all part of the set and setting. Just as a stage set changes the way we think about the actors in a play, the set and setting in which we drink helps to determine how we act while we are drinking and afterward.

The set is our state of mind—the "why" we are drinking and our expectations of alcohol. The setting is where we are drinking and with whom. Are we drinking alone in a dark bar after being fired? Are we drinking to forget? Are we hardly noticing that we're sipping a glass of wine with dinner, the same glass we routinely take? Are we pouring the bubbly to celebrate the great victory? Are we chugalugging to impress someone at a beer bust? The set and setting, the reason we're drinking, the emotions we bring to the first sip, the feelings we're enjoying or trying to hide—all these factors play a role in our emotional and behavioral responses to alcohol, and ultimately, in our physical responses as well. For example, a given amount of alcohol will have one effect on a group of fraternity brothers quaffing beer to celebrate the end of the semester, and quite another on a couple sipping spirits or wine during a romantic dinner. The amount of ethyl alcohol is the same, but the expectations, and thus the likely reactions, are quite different.

Which States Like Beer the Most?

NEVADA IS THE most beer-loving of the states, with residents quaffing 35.1 gallons of malt beverages per capita in 1994. Second place goes to New Hampshire, where 31.0 gallons per person were sipped in 1994. The District of Columbia is in third place at 28.7 gallons per capita, followed by Texas and Wisconsin, tied for fourth place at 28.3 gallons apiece. Utah is the least beer-loving of the states, with only 12.9 gallons per capita consumed in 1994.

How about Distilled Spirits?

ACCORDING TO STATISTICS published by the Distilled Spirits Council of the United States, New Hampshirites are the fondest of liquor, imbibing 4.08 gallons per capita in 1994. Once again Utah comes in last, its residents drinking only 0.71 gallons apiece in 1994.

And Wine?

WINES & VINES MAGAZINE ranked the fifty states and the District of Columbia according to their fondness for wine in 1994. First place went to the District of Columbia, home to the White House, Congress, and many embassies, where 4.9 gallons per capita are consumed every year. That's ten times as much per

continued

capita as Mississippi, the state least interested in wine, where residents drank only 0.49 gallons per capita in the same year.³

Our ongoing love affair with foreign wines contributes to the trade deficit. Between 1985 and 1994 we imported $9,896,092 worth of wine, but exported only $1,112,203 worth, thus adding $8,783,889 to the national deficit.⁴ Our favorite source of foreign wine is Italy: we imported 29,236,000 gallons from that country in 1994. Other favored sources include France, Chile, Spain, Australia, and Germany.⁵

THE HANGOVER AND "AFTER HANGOVER"

Perhaps one of alcohol's best known physiologic effects is the hangover, that pounding headache, dry mouth, dizziness, weakness, and general "blah" feeling that strikes the morning after overindulgence. It really doesn't matter what kind of alcoholic beverage you consume, or whether you switch from one drink to another—if you consume too much, you'll probably get a hangover. The first remedy for hangovers was undoubtedly devised soon after prehistoric man began drinking. Countless cures have been tried through the ages, including drinking sauerkraut juice, eating cabbage or persimmons, swallowing various B vitamins, sniffing oxygen from a tank, and gargling with a mixture of garlic and oil after rubbing butter on the forehead. These are interesting ideas, but they don't really work. Aspirin can dull the pain of a hangover headache and caffeinated beverages can provide a temporary "lift," but the only sure way to cure a hangover is to refrain from drinking to excess in the first place.

As if the hangover were not enough, alcohol can also cause an "after hangover." Like medicines and other drugs, alcohol can produce what is known as the "rebound effect." Many of us are familiar with caffeine rebound: A cup of coffee gives us a lift, but eventually the body metabolizes the coffee's caffeine and we start to feel low and jittery; we need another cup of coffee. Likewise, the "high" of cocaine and other uppers eventually fades away, leaving one feeling lower than ever. That's the rebound effect.

Alcohol has its own rebound effect. It initially relaxes us because it's a depressant. But when the sedative effect wears off, the brain and nervous system can become hyperactive. The after-hangover rebound may wake you up at night or prompt you to down another drink in a hurry, searching for calm. Unfortunately, doing so only prolongs the cycle of ups and downs.

ALCOHOL AND NUTRITION

Alcohol provides a small but significant percent of the total daily calories ingested by the average American—some 4.5%. (This figure is determined by averaging the food and alcohol intakes of all Americans, whether old or young, drinkers or nondrinkers.) Among adults who drink, the figure rises to 10 percent, and can be over 50 percent in heavy drinkers.[6]

Although wine, beer, and distilled spirits are made from fruits and grains, many of which are packed with nutrients, alcoholic beverages are not nutritional standouts. Depending upon the drink you consume, you'll get various (but invariably small) amounts of B vitamins, potassium, calcium, magnesium, and other vitamins and minerals, plus calories. Alcohol itself contains no fat or cholesterol, although certain drinks made with cream or other fatty ingredients certainly do. Generally speaking, beer is the most nutritious of alcoholic beverages, but even a quart of beer does not provide a significant portion of the Recommended Dietary Allowance for any nutrient.

However, alcoholic beverages do contain a number of beneficial phytochemicals. One of these is resveratrol, an antifungal compound found in grape skins that may lower cholesterol. Although some have speculated that wine's "healthy heart" properties may be due to resveratrol and other phytochemicals, the best available evidence suggests that ethyl alcohol itself deserves the credit. *Caution: Some wines contain sulfites and histamines, both of which can cause allergic reactions in susceptible people.*

ALCOHOL AND THE WAISTLINE

We usually think of alcohol as being fattening. After all, men who drink beer on the weekends tend to develop beer bellies, so alcohol must be a diet buster. Although some early studies supported the idea that alcohol was bad for the waistline, newer studies are disputing

35

these earlier findings, and are even suggesting that "proper" drinking *may* help to keep one slim.

First a few facts: Although alcohol contains no fat, it does have calories. One gram of alcohol contains approximately 7 calories (compared to 9 calories per gram of fat and 4 calories per gram of carbohydrate or protein). Clearly, drinking a lot of alcoholic beverages will push your calorie count up and your waistline out—just as you'll pack on the pounds if you eat too many calories from cookies, ice cream, or any source.

A 1994 project headed by William Rumpler, Ph.D., of the U.S. Department of Agriculture's Human Nutrition Research Center,[7] found that consuming moderate amounts of alcohol did not cause weight gain, and did not lead to an excess of body fat. In fact, some people developed healthier lean tissue-to-body fat profiles while drinking moderate amounts of alcohol. Although a great deal of research remains to be done, Dr. Rumpler believes that alcohol may help the body to regulate appetite.

Several papers appearing in the *Journal of the American College of Nutrition*[8] and the *American Journal of Clinical Nutrition*[9] have also suggested that moderate alcohol consumption does not make one obese. One researcher who studied sixteen young females who drank socially found that alcohol consumption increased their energy expenditure (calories burned) at rest.[10] The alcohol may, in effect, have slightly increased their metabolisms, causing them to burn more calories at all times. These findings echo those of a previous study, reported in the *American Journal of Public Health,* which found that drinking alcohol may lead to a slight increase in the resting metabolic rate.[11] (In all fairness, it should be noted that other studies have found that alcohol had no effect on resting metabolism in men, and actually slowed it in women.[12])

Why have some studies found that moderate alcohol consumption does not make one fat, while others say it does? Why do some report that it raises the resting metabolic rate, but others claim the opposite? There are many possible reasons. Some studies do not factor in the effects of smoking and lifestyle. Others fail to control for race. (Racial heritage may or may not turn out to be important, but at least one study found that White men and Black men had different weight-related responses to alcohol.[13]) The way people drink may also influence alcohol's effect on the waistline. New information taken from the National Heart, Lung and Blood Institute's study of 3,616 men and 2,141 women suggests that those who drink regularly, but only relatively small amounts each time, actually have lower body weights than those who drink a lot at once, or don't drink at all.[14]

The issue will undoubtedly be subject to continued debate.

WHAT'S NEXT

We've taken a quick look at alcohol's effects on the body, mind, and blood. Now that we know the "hows" and "whys" of alcohol in general, let's see how it can protect us from heart disease, stroke, the ravages of stress, and other problems.

CHAPTER FOUR

How Alcohol Protects the Heart

MANY PEOPLE HAVE cut back on fatty foods and are carefully monitoring their cholesterol levels, hoping to avoid a heart attack. It seems as if we've been concerned about clogged arteries forever, but the heart disease epidemic is actually a relatively modern problem. People living just one hundred years ago most likely worried more about succumbing to a ruptured appendix, tuberculosis, or pneumonia than a heart attack. Heart disease did not even appear on the "Top Ten Killer Disease" list until the twentieth century, but today it is the number-one killer in the United States. Despite tremendous advances in the medical and surgical treatment of this disease, in this year alone 1.5 million Americans will suffer heart attacks this year—and half a million will die of heart disease. There are 6.3 million living Americans who have had chest pain (angina pectoris), heart attacks, or both. And it's likely that heart disease will claim the lives of half of all Americans living today.

The idea that our hearts can suddenly stop pumping blood is terrifying. The warning pain that *may* strike sends many into a panic. So does the shortness of breath, fatigue, and "heaviness" in the chest that can herald a heart in distress. But in many cases there are no symptoms at all. The fatal heart attack that seems to come from nowhere is the only symptom.

Physicians have many tools designed to keep the heart healthy, including medicines that lower cholesterol, improve the flow of blood to the heart muscle, strengthen a heart weakened by previous attacks, and dissolve the blood clots that can trigger an attack. They can also perform a myriad of surgical techniques to keep things flowing smoothly.

ANOTHER MEDICINE FOR THE AILING HEART

Physicians also have another medicine for the heart, one that has largely been overlooked in recent years: moderate amounts of alcohol. The research suggests that there is a positive correlation between moderate alcohol intake and a reduced rate of heart disease. In other words, drinking in moderation can reduce your risk of having a heart attack. The studies have found:

- A decrease in coronary heart disease among 7,705 Japanese men living in Hawaii as their mean daily alcohol intake increased from 0 to 31.5 grams of alcohol a day. In other words, the men who drank moderate or heavy amounts of alcohol had *less* heart disease than those who drank little or none.[1]
- A drop in heart attacks among 1,505 Scottish men with high blood pressure who drank moderately.[2]
- A significantly lower risk of heart disease among 568 married White males who consumed four standard drinks daily versus those who did not.[3]
- Lower death rates from cardiovascular disease among 1,422 male civil servants who drank 34 grams of alcohol per day. This study, conducted over a ten-year period, found that nondrinkers were more likely to die from heart disease than were the imbibers.[4]
- Fewer heart attacks among 11,121 Yugoslavian men ages 35 to 60 who drank daily, as compared to occasional drinkers.[5]
- Lower rates of coronary heart disease and cardiovascular disease among 1,832 White males in Chicago who consumed 1–4 drinks per day.[6]

And the famous Framingham study found that those who drank 1.7–3.4 drinks per day had the lowest rate of coronary heart disease in the test group.[7] These are but a few of the many well-documented studies, conducted by respected researchers around the world, which show that small to moderate amounts of alcohol can have a protective effect upon the heart.

All in all, the results of many scientifically valid studies, conducted at research centers in many parts of the world and reported in prestigious medical journals, suggest that light to moderate consumption of wine, beer, or spirits can reduce the risk of suffering or dying from a heart attack.

A Time-Tested Remedy

THE IDEA THAT alcohol can have a beneficial effect on the heart is not new. Dr. Herberden, who in 1786 was the first to describe the chest pain (angina pectoris) that often warns of heart disease, also prescribed wine or spirits as a medicine for what was then a relatively new disease. And as late as 1951, the author of a noted book on heart disease described alcohol as "the most effective drug after nitrites" for the heart.[8]

HOW DOES MODERATE ALCOHOL CONSUMPTION AID THE HEART?

Several risk factors are known to increase the risk of heart disease. They are:

- High blood cholesterol
- Stress
- High blood pressure (hypertension)
- High blood fats (elevated triglycerides)
- Obesity
- Lack of exercise
- Cigarette smoking
- Diabetes
- Genetics

Having one or more of these risk factors does not mean that you will have a heart attack, but the unhappy odds do increase as the risk factors mount. Fortunately, small to moderate amounts of alcohol help to take the sting out of three of the risk factors, including stress, high blood pressure, and the single most deadly of them all: elevated cholesterol.

High blood cholesterol—Extensive studies have shown that small to medium amounts of alcohol moderate the number-one risk factor for heart disease by increasing the "good" HDL cholesterol that protects against heart disease, while possibly lowering the "bad" LDL cholesterol that harms the heart.

Stress—Moderate amounts of alcohol reduce the dangers of heart disease by relieving stress. Alcohol helps directly by reducing one's stress level, and indirectly by reducing the stress-related spasms of the coronary arteries that can halt the flow of blood through them. (We'll discuss the rocket scientist study and others that have linked stress to heart disease shortly.)

High blood pressure—Taken in small to moderate amounts, alcohol may lower blood pressure. *Caution: Chronic intake of high levels of alcohol may lead to elevations in blood pressure and increase the risk of heart disease.*

In addition, alcohol can help to protect against both heart disease and stroke by "thinning" the blood. Alcohol makes the platelets in the blood less sticky, and therefore less likely to clump together and trigger a heart attack or stroke by blocking the arteries feeding the heart muscle or the brain. Although the phenomenon of "stickiness" is not an independent risk factor for heart disease, preventing unnecessary clots is a helpful measure. Now let's take a closer look at the ways in which moderate consumption of alcohol helps to guard against cholesterol, stress, and high blood pressure.

Alcohol and Cholesterol

We commonly speak about cholesterol as if it were a single, evil entity. However, cholesterol is actually packaged in different forms inside the body by the liver. These cholesterol-containing "packages," called lipoproteins, also contain protein and fat. As far as heart disease is concerned, the two most important cholesterol packages are the high-density lipoprotein (HDL) and the low-density lipoprotein (LDL).

HDL is called the "good" cholesterol because it travels through the bloodstream scavenging cholesterol from the arteries, pulling it off the arterial walls, and taking it to the liver for disposal. The HDL level is inversely proportional to the risk of heart disease. This means that the higher the HDL (up to a point), the lower the risk of heart disease. But as HDL levels fall, the risk of heart disease rises. (The National Cholesterol Education Program says that an HDL of less than 35 is an independent risk factor for coronary heart disease. Most doctors agree that the HDL should be at least 45 for optimal heart health.)

LDL is known as the "bad" cholesterol because it carries cholesterol to the artery walls, where it can stick and form blockages. We need some LDL, but too much can encourage heart disease, which is why lower levels of this "bad" cholesterol are considered better for the heart. An LDL of 100 or less is felt to be safe.

Many studies looking at large groups of people have found a link between the "good" HDL and alcohol consumption.[9] That is, those who consume alcohol tend to have higher HDLs than those who do not. These findings have been repeated in experimental studies in which some people were asked to drink measured amounts of alcohol, while others were not. When the HDL levels of the drinkers and non-drinkers were compared, it was found that it only takes a few weeks of moderate imbibing to increase the levels of the "good" cholesterol in the blood.

Not satisfied with simply knowing that moderate alcohol consumption can raise the "good" cholesterol, researchers have tried to determine how much of alcohol's protective effect upon the heart can be attributed to the increased HDL. Analysis of the 11,688 people in the "MR. FIT" study, the Honolulu Heart Study, and the LRC Follow-Up Study suggest that increases in HDL account for approximately half of alcohol's beneficial effects upon the heart.

ALCOHOL AND STRESS

In addition to raising the protective HDL, small to medium amounts of alcohol can also moderate the effects of stress, a phenomenon that has been firmly linked to heart disease for the past several decades.

Many physicians and lay people have long suspected that stress was related to heart disease, but the relationship was not seriously investigated until the 1960s, when young rocket scientists at Cape Kennedy began dying of heart disease at an alarming rate. Wondering whether or not the Russians were to blame, the government sent Robert Elliot, M.D., to investigate. After eliminating both the Russians and coronary heart disease as suspected causes, Dr. Elliot discovered that the real culprit was stress. It seems that despite the success of the space program, the budget-conscious government was continually laying people off. Not knowing if they would have their prized jobs tomorrow, these scientists were stressed. They feared that at any time they would lose

Helpful Guidelines for Heart Health

PHYSICIANS HAVE DEVISED two quick and easy ways to gauge your risk of heart disease. These tests are called the Coronary Artery Disease Risk Factors One and Two, or CADRF 1 and CADRF 2, for short. In order to calculate your CADRFs, you must first ask your doctor for the results of your latest blood tests. Ask for your total cholesterol, HDL and LDL figures.

To get the CADRF 1, divide your total cholesterol (TC) by your HDL. For example, if your TC is 250 and your HDL is 50, your CADRF 1 is 250/50 = 5. The lower the CADRF 1, the better.

For men, a CADRF 1 of 4.97 gives you an average risk of suffering from a heart attack. With a CADRF 1 of 3.43, however, you have only half the average risk. But, going the other way, if your CADRF 1 is 9.55 you have twice the risk, and the odds climb to three times the average if your CADRF 1 hits 23.39.

For women, the average risk of heart disease is found with a CADRF 1 of 4.44. The risk doubles at 7.05, and triples at 11.04. But it falls to half when the CADRF 1 drops to 3.27.

CADRF 2 compares the "good" and "bad" cholesterols. To determine your CADRF 2, divide your LDL by your HDL. For example, if your LDL is 210 and your HDL is 30, your CADRF 2 is 210/30 = 7. The lower the CADRF 2, the lower the risk of having a heart attack.

For men, a CADRF 2 of 3.55 gives an average risk. The risk doubles at 6.25 and triples at 7.99, but falls to only half at 1.00.

For women, 1.47 is the desirable CADRF 2, offering only half the average risk of heart disease. The risk becomes average at 3.22, twice the average at 5.03, and three times the average at 6.14.

When figuring your CADRFs, remember that you want to be better than average, for the average American with the average risk factors has the average heart attack.

Stress and Cholesterol

STRESS HARMS THE heart by raising the blood pressure and increasing the levels of adrenalinlike substances called catecholamines. It also increases the risk of heart disease by elevating the levels of cholesterol in the blood. Numerous scientific studies have shown the relationship between stress and elevated cholesterol. If you stress people by throwing them into ice-cold water, for example, their cholesterol levels will rise. If you threaten them, if you tell them they're going be fired or they are going to have to take difficult tests, their cholesterol levels invariably will increase.

Years ago, studies of doctors, lawyers, and accountants showed that all three of these groups had elevated cholesterol levels because of poor dietary habits. However, even though they did not change their diets, the accountants' cholesterol levels went up even higher during tax season (as compared to those of the doctors and attorneys). The accountants were eating the same foods, but they were under additional stress, which caused the rise in cholesterol. Many studies have shown that a variety of stressful conditions can cause cholesterol levels to rise as much as 35 percent. Watching what you eat isn't enough: You must also reduce your stress levels in order to keep your cholesterol in check.

their livelihoods, as well as their identities as the best and the brightest. The stress was literally destroying their heart muscles and killing them.

This stress-heart disease link has been confirmed by many research studies. In one such study, laboratory rats were locked in a cage and forced to listen to a recording of cats chasing rats. The rats didn't know that they were listening to a recording; they thought a real cat was nearby, about to come after them. They were terribly stressed and fearful. Soon, they began dying from necroses of the heart (death of the heart muscle), just like the rocket scientists. Other lab rats, who did not have to listen to the recording, remained in good health.

Just as the link between stress and heart disease is well established, so is the relationship between alcohol and stress. As England's Dr. Thomas Stuttaford writes: "In moderate amounts, alcohol reduces anxiety, calms the emotions and thereby diminishes stress. Various experimental devices have been used to measure the effect of alcohol on a tense subject; not surprisingly it has been found to be useful when taken in small or moderate amounts. . . . Alcohol diminished tension, self-consciousness and depression . . ."[10]

We'll take a closer look at the relationship between alcohol and stress in the next chapter.

ALCOHOL AND BLOOD PRESSURE

If moderate alcohol consumption only increased the "good" HDL cholesterol and reduced the stress-induced heart damage, it would be considered a strong medicine. But it does more. Small to moderate amounts of alcohol can also lower blood pressure, a third heart disease risk factor.

Stress can increase the cardiac output by making the heart beat harder and faster. When we're stressed, the brain sends "red alert" messages to the sympathetic nervous system, which prompts the insides of the adrenal glands (the adrenal medullas) to pump out adrenalinelike substances. These substances increase the heart rate and the power with which the heart beats, sending the blood pressure soaring.

That's not all. When we're stressed, the hypothalamus, the "pilot" of the brain, tells the pituitary gland to release a hormone called ACTH (adrenalcorticotrophic hormone). ACTH directs the adrenal glands to put out a number of other hormones, including some forty different varieties of cortisone, plus aldosterone. These hormones cause the body to retain salt and water. Extra fluid and sodium in the body means that there's more fluid in the bloodstream, more fluid that has to be pumped through the body. This elevates blood pressure.

And there's more. With chronic stress, the blood vessels constrict, they "tighten up" and get smaller. With the "pipes" smaller, it's harder for the blood to flow through, which means that blood pressure goes up. To darken the picture even more, chronic stress changes the chemistry of the blood, making it more likely to clot. This means there's a greater chance that a clot will form and trigger a heart attack by getting stuck in a partially narrowed coronary artery.

It's a simple formula: Stress = greater output + greater resistance

+ more fluid = elevated blood pressure. Clearly, keeping stress levels low helps to reduce the risk of high blood pressure. And since alcohol in moderation reduces stress, alcohol may also lower blood pressure and reduce the risk of heart disease.

Caution: Long-term usage of larger amounts of alcohol can have the reverse effect, raising blood pressure. Always drink in moderation, if you drink at all. If you have any reason to suspect that your blood pressure is elevated, see your physician.

ALCOHOL AND THE BLOOD

Although having "sticky platelets" in the blood is not an independent risk factor for coronary heart disease, blood clots are a major contributor to this often fatal condition. A clot that forms in or drifts into an already-narrowed coronary artery can trigger a sudden, possibly fatal heart attack by stopping the flow of blood. In fact, studies have shown that the risk of heart problems can be predicted by measuring the degree to which platelets in the blood will "stick" together and form blood clots (platelet aggregation).[11] The greater the tendency to "stick," the greater the odds of suffering a heart attack.

In 1987, researchers reported that platelets became less reactive if wine was consumed for as little as five weeks.[12] A 1990 study found that red wine could produce the same effect in as little as two weeks.[13] (White wine and diluted alcohol did not produce the same beneficial results.) Although long-term studies are needed, it seems that moderate amounts of alcohol are able to keep the platelets from becoming unnecessarily "sticky," thereby helping to prevent the unwanted blood clots that play such an important role in heart disease.

WINE, BEER, AND LIQUOR ARE EQUALLY GOOD FOR THE HEART

Some have suggested that wine might be better for the heart than beer or liquor because it contains fungicides, anthocyanins, tannins, quercetin, resveratrol, and other phytochemicals. It's true that these substances have antioxidant and other protective effects, and that many studies have praised wine's cardioprotective prowess. However:

- As the authors of a report appearing in 1991 in the *British Medical Journal* pointed out, "An apparent greater protection from wine compared with other alcoholic beverages could arise from the fact that moderate drinkers of wine tend to be of higher social class than non-drinkers. That alone is associated with lower risk."[14] In other words, the people who choose to drink wine may be at lower risk for coronary heart disease to begin with.
- Some studies have praised wine over beer or liquor. But others have come to different conclusions. For example, the authors of a 1991 study titled "Prospective Study of Alcohol Consumption and Risk of Coronary Disease in Men"[15] concluded that liquor had the strongest effects. And back in 1977, the authors of a study appearing in the prestigious *New England Journal of Medicine* had singled out beer.[16]

The bulk of the scientific evidence suggests that it doesn't matter what type of alcoholic beverage is consumed. In a 1986 paper appearing in the *American Journal of Cardiology,* noted alcohol researcher Arthur Klatsky of the Kaiser Permanente Medical Center and his coauthors asserted that "The unimportant role of beverage type suggests that reduced [coronary heart disease] risk is associated either with ethyl alcohol itself or with some other trait present among persons who consume any type of alcoholic beverage."[17] In other words, it doesn't seem to matter whether one consumes beer, wine, or spirits. And in a 1995 article appearing in the *American Journal of Clinical Nutrition,*[18] the authors referred to "the consistent finding from observational studies that consumption of all types of alcoholic beverages is associated with lower rates" of coronary heart disease. This suggests that ethyl alcohol itself is the key factor. The most recent word on the subject, from researchers at Harvard and other prestigious institutions, was published in the *British Medical Journal* in March of 1996. After reviewing twenty-five previously published studies on alcohol and the risk of coronary artery disease, the scientists concluded that "The evidence suggests that all alcoholic drinks are linked with lower risk, so that much of the benefit is from alcohol rather than other components of each type of drink."[19]

As far as heart health is concerned, it appears that all alcoholic beverages are equally beneficial.

A large number of scientifically valid studies conducted at prestigious medical centers have demonstrated that small to medium amounts of alcohol can have a protective effect on the heart, by guarding against coronary heart disease, the number-one killer disease in the United States today. As the International Life Sciences Institute explains, "A moderate intake of alcohol in the form of beer, wine, or spirits apparently protects by 10–70%" against fatal and nonfatal heart attacks.[20]

In the words of Gary Friedman, M.D., and Arthur Klatsky, M.D., two of the nation's foremost experts on alcohol and health, "There now seems little doubt that alcohol exerts a protective effect against coronary heart disease. Most large-scale studies have shown that people who consume one or two drinks a day have fewer coronary events than abstainers."[21]

Even the American Heart Association, a mainstream health organization with no reason to favor alcohol, agrees, saying: "There is no evidence, however, that moderate long-term use of alcohol increases the risk of coronary heart disease (heart attack). There is evidence that moderate intake may be beneficial."[22]

For a detailed review of the scientific literature examining the beneficial effects of alcohol on the heart, including studies published in prestigious journals such as the *Journal of the American Medical Association, Lancet, Annals of Internal Medicine,* the *American Journal of Epidemiology,* the *American Journal of Cardiology* and the *British Medical Journal,* see Appendix I.

If you don't already drink alcohol, don't start just to get the heart-health benefits. And if you do drink, don't increase your consumption. As you'll see in Chapter 8, there are many ways to strengthen your heart without alcohol.

CHAPTER FIVE

Reducing the Risk of Stroke

STROKE! OUR IMAGES of the disease are frightening: A sudden, blinding pain that strikes from within the head. A sledgehammer blow that drives us to our knees, forever robbing us of our ability to walk, talk, move our arms, or even use a fork.

The third leading killer disease in the United States, stroke is also the number-one cause of disability among adults. This year 550,000 Americans will have a stroke—more than one every single minute of every single day. Presidents Woodrow Wilson and Franklin Roosevelt both suffered strokes while in office. President Wilson was able to finish out his term, but the stroke cut short both Roosevelt's term and his life.

My grandfather was also a victim of stroke, falling to a massive one when he was in his early seventies. This strong man was a former boxer who was known for knocking opponents to the ground with a single punch and who later became a fruit broker who easily slung several fifty-pound boxes of fruit onto his shoulders, sometimes carrying them for blocks. But when an artery in his brain burst, he crumpled helplessly to the floor. The last time I saw him alive he was lying in a hospital bed in a coma.

WHAT IS A STROKE?

Even more than the rest of the body, the brain needs oxygen. Oxygen-rich blood is supplied to the brain through a network of arteries that nourish each and every cell in our gray matter. But if the flow of blood is cut off, oxygen-starved brain cells die. That's a stroke.

In a more technical vein, a stroke can be described as a sudden disturbance in blood flow to a part of the brain, leading to temporary or permanent damage. What kind of damage, and how severe it is, depends upon which part of the brain was injured, and to what extent. If, for example, cells in the part of the brain controlling speech are damaged, you may have difficulty speaking—to the point of being completely unable to utter coherent sounds.

Although symptoms of a stroke vary greatly from person to person, difficulty in speaking, a sudden heaviness or numbness in an arm or leg, inability to control movement, visual disturbances, nausea, vomiting, temporary amnesia, headaches, dizziness, and confusion are common. A smaller number of stroke victims will lose consciousness.

Some people are "lucky" enough to suffer from small strokes that serve as warnings, prompting them to get medical attention immediately. For others, the first sign of trouble is a major stroke that is either fatal or leaves them seriously incapacitated.

Although people age sixty and up are at a greater risk of stroke than younger folks, strokes can happen at any age. Besides age, the other risk factors for stroke include:

- high blood pressure (hypertension)—elevated blood pressure is the number-one risk factor for stroke. Even mild hypertension can increase the risk
- coronary artery disease—the cholesterol, blood fats, and other factors that can clog arteries in the heart, or make them brittle and likely to rupture, can do the same to arteries in the brain
- other forms of heart disease—congestive heart disease, atrial fibrillation, and other forms of heart disease may lead to the formation of blood clots that can move through the bloodstream to the smaller cerebral arteries and possibly get stuck, precipitating a stroke
- Transient Ischemic Attacks (TIAs)—people who have had these "baby strokes" are 9.5 times more likely to suffer a major stroke than others of the same sex and age who have not been struck by TIAs.
- smoking—nicotine, carbon monoxide, and other substances in cigarette smoke are believed to damage the circulatory system and increase the risk of stroke
- prior strokes—the risk of suffering a stroke is greater in those who have already had them than it is in those who have not
- diabetes mellitus—diabetes slowly damages and plugs up arteries.

It also makes the blood more "sticky," increasing the odds that a clot will form and lodge in an artery in the brain
- a family history of stroke
- Obesity—obesity likely leads to increased fat in the blood, encouraging plugged arteries and "thicker" blood
- physical inactivity—the more physically active you are, the less the likelihood that your blood will form unnecessary and dangerous clots
- sex—men are at higher risk of stroke than are women

Excessive alcohol consumption is also a major risk factor for stroke.

TWO MAJOR "TYPES" OF STROKE

Doctors describe strokes as *cerebral infarctions, intracerebral hemorrhages,* or *subarachnoid hemorrhages,* but it's simpler to think of them as "blockage strokes" and "rupture strokes."

A blockage stroke is almost the same thing as a heart attack, but it happens in the brain. Just as the heart depends on fresh blood flowing through the coronary arteries, the brain draws nourishment from oxygen-rich blood in the cerebral (brain) arteries. If the blood stops circulating because an artery is blocked, brain cells "downstream" of the blockage die. Blockage strokes may be caused by the narrowing or complete clogging of a cerebral artery *(cerebral thrombosis).* The cholesterol, fat, and other factors that gum up the coronary arteries are the same villains that cause blockage strokes. Blockages may also be caused by a free-floating particle that lodges in a brain artery *(cerebral embolism),* halting the flow of blood. The embolism is typically caused by a blood clot that travels easily through larger, wider arteries, then gets stuck when the bloodstream sweeps it into a smaller and narrower artery. The clot may originate in the brain, or it could float through the bloodstream from the heart, legs, or another part of the body.

Rupture strokes are, in a sense, the opposite of blockage strokes. Instead of a lack of blood, there's too much blood in a part of the brain. This happens when a cerebral vessel "breaks" and blood pours into the brain tissue, or in the area between the brain and skull, just like water spewing from a broken fire hydrant. The excess fluid in the area around the break can put intense pressure on the nearby brain cells, damaging or killing them. The body tries to repair the break, just as it does a cut in the finger. If successful, the body's self-repair mechanisms may hold damage to a minimum. If not, the results can be disastrous.

Why do brain arteries rupture? In some cases a buildup of cholesterol and fat weakens the arteries from the inside out. In other cases, a little balloonlike "out pouching" of an artery called an *aneurysm* develops. If the "balloon" bursts, blood pours from the artery into the surrounding brain tissue, "drowning" the brain cells.

Whether a blockage stroke or a rupture stroke, a disturbance in blood flow through the brain can cause anything from mild and temporary speech difficulties to serious disability or death.

How Alcohol Can Help to Reduce the Risk of Stroke

Alcohol reduces the risk of blockage strokes in much the same way that it works against coronary heart disease. Remember, blockage strokes are "clogged pipe" problems, just like the heart attacks caused by coronary heart disease. Preventing blockage strokes is simply a matter of keeping the cerebral arteries open and the blood flowing freely. Small to moderate amounts of alcohol can help to do this by:

- increasing the levels of the helpful HDL cholesterol
- lessening the odds that anything will stick to the walls of the brain arteries
- "thinning" the blood, thereby reducing the risk that a blood clot will form, lodge in a cerebral artery, and stop the flow of blood
- reducing the odds of a sudden spasm of the smooth muscle surrounding the cerebral arteries

What the Medical Literature Has to Say about Alcohol and Stroke

Common wisdom has long held that drinking alcohol causes strokes. While it is true that excessive or binge drinking can trigger a brain accident, and that overindulgence can increase the risk of stroke by pushing up blood pressure, the scientific evidence suggests that alcohol is not the villain it's been made out to be.

Also Known As

Brain attack—Some researchers refer to strokes as "brain attacks," drawing on the comparison between heart attacks and "blockage" strokes (both of which are caused by clogged or damaged arteries).

Cerebral infarct—The word "infarct" comes from the French, meaning "to stuff." Whether brain tissue is "stuffed" with blood in a "rupture" stroke or the artery is stuffed and blocked in a "blockage" stroke, the result can be deadly.

Cerebrovascular accident (CVA)—"Cerebro" refers to the brain, and "vascular" to the arteries and veins supplying blood to the gray matter. Thus, a cerebrovascular accident is a problem with the plumbing in the brain, better known as a stroke.

Ischemia—a decreased supply of blood to a body tissue or organ.

Little strokes—These are relatively minor strokes that produce minimal and often very brief damage. Indeed, they can be so "small" that the victim doesn't realize what has happened. Instead, he or she may attribute the sudden dizziness or nausea to the flu. Winston Churchill, who led Great Britain through World War II, suffered from a series of small strokes during the height of that worldwide conflict.

Transient ischemic attack (TIA)—a brief disturbance in the blood supply to a part of the brain. Often lasting for only a few minutes, a TIA may produce symptoms such as dizziness, weakness, visual disturbances, and unconsciousness. Some 36 percent of those who have had a TIA will later suffer from a stroke.

Dry stroke—an ischemic or "blockage" stroke. It's called a "dry" stroke because the blood flow "dries up" beyond the blockage.

Wet stroke—a hemorrhagic or "rupture" stroke in which blood leaks from a blood vessel into the brain

1 Drink = 10 Grams Alcohol

SOME OF THE alcohol/health studies refer to "drinks," others to grams of alcohol. A single drink is generally defined as:

- a glass of wine (about 5 ounces of fluid), or
- a can of beer (about 12 ounces of fluid), or
- 1.5 ounces spirits (equal to a shot of whiskey)

The glass of wine, can of beer, and serving of spirits are equivalent in that they all contain the same amount of alcohol (about 10–12 grams, or ½ ounce).

Many researchers have looked into the relationship between alcohol consumption and stroke. Unlike the heart/alcohol studies, which show a clear and strong indication of alcohol's heart benefits at low to moderate levels of consumption, the stroke/alcohol studies provide weaker, sometimes confusing evidence. It is clear, however, that:

- several studies point to a small measure of protection against blockage strokes offered by light to moderate drinking
- more than a couple of drinks a day increases the risk of rupture strokes
- binge drinking likely increases the risk of stroke

You would expect light to moderate consumption of alcohol to protect against blockage strokes, which are similar to coronary heart disease. The scientific evidence suggests that this may be true, and that in any case, light to moderate consumption does *not* increase the risk. As for rupture strokes, it appears that blood pressure elevations and possibly other factors associated with habitual alcohol consumption can increase the risk of these. Let's take a closer look at the issue by reviewing selected studies from the medical literature.

This 1988 case-controlled study published in the *International Jour-*

nal of Epidemiology[1] found that light drinkers were less likely to suffer from strokes than were abstainers.

STUDY SUMMARY: The researchers looked at alcohol consumption, as well as the blood and biologic markers of alcohol intake in people admitted to the hospital for strokes. These subjects were compared to community-based controls taken from an occupational screening survey. RESULTS: Although heavy drinking was associated with an increased risk of stroke, lighter drinkers who consumed less than 30 units per week were less likely to suffer strokes than those who abstained.

A large-scale study published the same year in the *New England Journal of Medicine*[2] also found that moderate consumption of alcohol offered protection against stroke.

STUDY SUMMARY: 87,526 female nurses ranging in age from 34–59 were asked to report their consumption of alcohol on a dietary questionnaire. The women were followed until 1984, and the data was analyzed. RESULTS: The researchers found that drinking light to moderate amounts of alcohol offered protection against ischemic (blockage) strokes. Women drinking 14 grams of alcohol per day had a relative risk of 0.3, well below the relative risk of 1.0 for the nondrinkers. (However, the odds of suffering a hemorrhagic stroke increased among drinkers.)

Swiss researchers looked into the brain-protective effects of alcohol in this 1990 study published in *Stroke*.[3] They found that moderate alcohol consumption protected against blockages of the main arteries leading to the brain.

STUDY SUMMARY: 261 patients over the age of fifty and suffering from their first ischemic strokes were studied. These people were suffering from carotid atherosclerosis, or "hardening" of the carotid arteries, which run along the sides of the neck to supply fresh blood to the brain. RESULTS: After gathering information on the patients' drinking patterns, the researchers found that "light to moderate consumption of alcohol is the first factor to be inversely associated with extra-cranial carotid atherosclerosis in symptomatic patients with cerebrovascular disease." In other words, small amounts of alcohol reduced their risk of developing "hardening" of the carotid arteries.

In this interesting study presented in the *American Journal of Medicine,*[4] alcohol was found to reduce the risk of both blockage and rupture strokes in light drinkers. That's unusual, for most studies find that alcohol only protects against blockage strokes.

STUDY SUMMARY: 621 stroke patients and 573 controls were enrolled in this case-controlled study. The stroke victims were then divided according to whether they had suffered a subarachnoid hemorrhage, an intracerebral hemorrhage, or cerebral infarction. RESULTS: The relative risks for all three types of stroke were lower in light to moderate drinkers. The study's authors noted that low levels of alcohol consumption seem to have a protective effect on the arteries in the brain, but warned that heavy drinking is a risk factor for stroke.

As was the case with heart disease, the studies showing that alcohol can help prevent blockage strokes were criticized on the grounds that they did not properly distinguish between lifelong abstainers and those who had once been drinkers but had given it up completely. Even though the studies reported that light to moderate drinkers were at lower risk than abstainers, critics argued that the results were skewed because sick former drinkers were grouped together with the lifelong teetotalers. The ones who drank themselves sick, they said, made the "abstainers" group look sicker than it would have been if it only included true nondrinkers. If you excluded the "sick quitters," the argument ran, the abstaining groups would be healthier overall, and would have risk factors comparable to the light to moderate drinkers. In other words, taking the sick former drinkers out of the "never drink" group would erase the statistical benefits of light imbibing. A 1993 study presented in *Stroke*[5] dealt with that issue.

STUDY SUMMARY: 364 stroke victims were matched for age and sex with 364 controls. Their current and past drinking habits were examined. RESULTS: "Stroke patients were more likely to have been lifelong abstainers from alcohol than were the control subjects." And "no relation was found between stroke and current non-drinkers." In other words, lifetime "abstention from alcohol is associated with an increased risk of stroke," and moderate drinking does offer protection.

Some people enjoy a relatively small and regular amount of wine, beer, or liquor every day, week, or month. Binge drinkers, however, consume a lot of alcohol in brief periods of time. Does it matter if one is a steady drinker or a binge drinker? Two researchers from the neurology department of Finland's University of Helsinki looked into the way differing patterns of alcohol consumption affected the risk of stroke in men. The results of this study, which dealt with blockage strokes, were published in *Stroke*[6] in 1993.

STUDY SUMMARY: Slightly over 300 young and middle-aged men were included in this case-controlled study, with about half serving as controls. The men were classified as nondrinkers, light-to-moderate drinkers (150 grams of alcohol a week or less), moderate drinkers (up to 300 grams per week) or heavy drinkers (more than 300 grams per week). They were also designated as "regular" drinkers if they consumed daily or almost daily, and "irregular" drinkers if they drank up to three times a week. The point of dividing "regular" and "irregular" drinkers was to determine if drinking patterns played a role in preventing (or triggering) strokes. This would enable the researchers to determine if (1) alcohol helped prevent ischemic strokes, and if (2) regular drinking was more beneficial than sporadic drinking. RESULTS: Light-to-moderate drinkers enjoyed a measure of protection from ischemic strokes, especially "if the consumption of alcohol is regular and evenly distributed throughout the week . . ." (*Heavy* drinking, however, was found to be a risk factor for blockage stroke.)

For a look at more alcohol/stroke studies, see Appendix 2.

IN CONCLUSION

There's good news and there's bad news. First the bad. Drinking can increase the risk of suffering a rupture stroke, especially habitual consumption. We don't know exactly where the cutoff point is, but one is playing a risky game of odds when he or she enjoys more than a drink or two a day. Binge drinking is also a losing proposition, with a small body of scientific evidence suggesting that alternating periods of heavy drinking with periods of abstention may be linked to an increase in stroke.

And now for the good news. A large amount of evidence suggests that light to moderate consumption of alcoholic beverages reduces the risk of blockage strokes in many people. As one researcher puts it,

"Lighter drinking habits appear to offer significant protection against . . . ischemic strokes."[7]

And the *overall* effect of light to moderate drinking on stroke (blockage plus rupture) is positive, lowering the risk somewhat. Fortunately, it is also possible to reduce the risk of stroke in many ways without drinking alcohol, as you'll see in Chapter 8.

CHAPTER SIX

Alcohol Fights Stress

WE HUMAN BEINGS are, in many ways, generalists. That is, we don't have a specific way of responding to being chased by a lion, another specialized reaction to being fired, a unique method for getting through a divorce, and yet a fourth defense for dealing with incompetent and uncaring clerks. Instead, we have a single, all-purpose response to things that annoy, harass, frighten, terrify, or otherwise stress us. This single defensive mechanism is called the "fight or flight response."

We're generalists, but the problems that daily bombard us are specific: An angry dog is running toward us, the third quarter totals were low, we failed the certification test, the jerk in the red car cuts us off, the bank refuses to loan the money, the clerk shortchanges us a dollar. The problems vary but our reaction is always the same: We perceive everything as a danger, and react accordingly.

Every time these real or imagined dangers arise, the brain sets in motion an intricate series of biochemical and electrical events that prepare the body to either fight for life or run away. A part of the brain called the hypothalamus sends a chemical messenger known as ACTH[1] down to the adrenal glands, one of which sits atop each of the two kidneys. The adrenals, which are each about the size of a thumb, immediately begin pumping out large quantities of adrenaline[2] and other powerful substances that kick the body into high gear. In no time at all:

- the heart beats faster and more vigorously, sending blood coursing through arteries and veins
- respiration speeds up to get more oxygen into the body

- the numbers of oxygen-carrying red blood cells increases, carrying the extra oxygen in the lungs to every part of the body
- more white blood cells, the mainstay of the immune system, appear in the bloodstream, ready to grapple with any "germs" that may enter through breaks in the skin, or that have already made their way into the body
- muscle tension and strength increase
- the pupils of the eyes dilate to improve vision
- blood sugar shoots up to make more energy available
- sweating increases to throw off the excess heat generated by these sudden, jarring changes in body chemistry

. . . and the body otherwise prepares for the fight of its life, or to get the heck out of harm's way. Meanwhile, any body function that gets in the way of fighting or running, such as digesting food, is shut down. (That's why some people vomit under stress—the body is simply getting rid of a distraction.)

CAN WE OVERDO THE FIGHT-OR-FLIGHT RESPONSE?

The fight-or-flight response has a hair trigger; it takes very little to set it off. That makes a lot of sense if life is fraught with danger. Imagine a caveman walking down the path when suddenly he hears a noise in the bush. BOOM! The fight-or-flight response is instantly triggered because there's no time to investigate, to analyze the noise, to figure out whether it's a huge man-eating lion or a little mouse hiding in that bush. It's safer to assume the worse and to be ready. If it was a tiger ready to pounce, the caveman was ready. But suppose it's just a mouse?

Our bodies are jolted every time the fight-or-flight response is triggered. Epinephrine, norepinephrine, catecholamine, and many other highly charged chemicals flood the body, shocking organs and systems. Blood and other substances are shuttled around the body as some organs are thrust into the spotlight, while others are shunted to the sidelines. The body practically wrenches itself upside down as it gears for action—then sees a mouse.

What's the harm? Well, the fight-or-flight response begins with the equivalent of a five-alarm siren wailing in the body. After a brief alarm reaction, the body enters into the stage of resistance. Not knowing if the danger will be brief or prolonged, the adrenal glands flood the body with many substances, including numerous varieties of cortisone hormones. That's good for people who really need to fight or run, but bad for those who don't. And most of the time, we trigger the response for nothing. We trigger it when we're yelled at by the boss, even though there's no one to punch and no place to flee. We trigger it when we argue with someone over politics or religion, when we fight over parking spaces or seats on the bus, and when we quarrel with our spouses.

Many of us are constantly in the fight-or-flight mode as we stew over problems and slights, large and small, real or imagined. Here are just a few of the things that can happen to those of us who see danger everywhere, all the time:

- the body's control mechanisms are thrown out of kilter by the constant flood of high-powered stress chemicals in the body
- blood sugar rises
- healing is inhibited
- the ability to manufacture protein decreases
- little by little, the immune system falters
- the bloodstream becomes "waterlogged" as the body retains sodium and water. With more fluid to pump, the heart must work harder and blood pressure rises. If this happens too often, blood pressure may become permanently elevated
- blood vessels are sensitized during fight-or-flight. This means that they'll constrict easily to raise blood pressure, which is important when facing real danger. But if the response is triggered too often, the blood pressure may remain permanently elevated
- the body needs a great deal of energy during the stage of resistance, so it "steals" proteins from muscles, organs, and other body tissue. That's a little like tearing down the walls of your house to get wood to burn in the furnace. A little bit of that is okay, but too much will leave you without a house.

All this explains why the stage of resistance eventually gives way to the stage of exhaustion. If the stress is too strong or lasts too long, the body's resources are eventually exhausted. Without the strength to deal with anything at all, let alone stress, you're easy prey for all kinds of disease and distress.

How dangerous is repeated stress? It can literally be deadly. In Chapter 4, I introduced the rocket scientists and laboratory rats who were literally stressed to death. The dangerous effects of stress on the human heart can be easily measured in a modern laboratory. If, for example, you hook people up to devices that monitor their hearts, then ask them to perform stressful tasks such as public speaking, you can "see" how their fear interferes with their hearts' ability to pump blood properly. The adverse effects of stress on the heart were demonstrated in a study published in the *Journal of the American Medical Association* in June of 1996.[3] One hundred twelve men and 14 women, all suffering from documented coronary artery disease, participated. The researchers were investigating mental stress and reduced blood flow to the heart. This is an important area of study, for mental stress simultaneously increases the heart's need for oxygen while cutting back on the supply. (That's a little like having to run a mile with a clamp squeezing your neck. You need more air, but can't get it.) The researchers found that the patients who suffered from a stress-related lack of blood to the heart were significantly more likely to suffer from fatal and nonfatal heart attacks.

Stress also increases the risk of heart disease and stroke by driving up both blood pressure and cholesterol.

STRESS AND DEPRESSION

Depression, a major "subset" of stress, has a powerful but negative influence on the immune system. Although the immune system is composed of various cells and tissues spread throughout the body, the entire system is controlled by the brain. There are, for example, receptors on the immune system's white blood cells that allow the brain to issue orders directly to these powerful immune-fighters.

The brain never hesitates to communicate with the rest of the body, even when the news is bad and the effect upon the health worse. Hundreds of years before Christ was born, the ancient Greek physician Hippocrates noted that depressed women were more likely to develop cancer of the breast or uterus than women who were not depressed. More recently, many studies have shown that the stress of depression weakens the immune system. For example, men whose wives have died generally become depressed and anxious, which is natural. Tests show that the number of immune-system cells in their bodies falls while they are grieving, and that their immune systems weaken in general.

Depression can strike the heart as lethally as it does the immune system. A 1991 study published in *Epidemiology* revealed that depressed people had a greater risk of fatal and nonfatal heart attacks

Diseases Caused or Made Worse by Stress

ACCORDING TO ARNOLD FOX, M.D., a noted internist and cardiologist practicing in Beverly Hills, California, stress can cause or worsen a long list of diseases, including cardiovascular disease, stroke, and diabetes. Stress also depresses the immune system, leaving us open to everything from colds to cancer. "That's why I tell my patients that the biggest killer in the United States is stress" he says. In fact, he calls stress "thought disease," and teaches his patients how to fight back by giving themselves a daily dose of enthusiasm, belief, love, forgiveness, and perseverance. He calls these the " Virtues," and feels that they are the best medicine for "thought disease."

than their nondepressed peers. And when you look at large populations, you see that as the sense of hopelessness increases, so do the rates of disease and death.

It's clear that stress is dangerous, and must be kept under control. (By the way, it's interesting to note that people who are legally insane have a lower incidence of stress-related diseases such as heart attacks, stroke, cancer, and diabetes. Apparently, they don't know when they're being stressed, so they don't suffer its adverse effects.)

ALCOHOL HELPS TO RELIEVE STRESS

Physicians have long prescribed a glass or two of alcohol to help their stressed patients. They weren't able to point to any stress/alcohol studies, but they knew that a little bit of alcohol helped many people suffering from stress or depression. They knew, as Dr. Thomas Stuttaford pointed out in Chapter 4, that moderate imbibing "diminished tension, self-consciousness and depression, and increased conviviality."[4]

Today, many hospitals rely on alcohol to relieve their patients' stress. One-third of a group of hospitals in sixty-five major United States cities reported that they sometimes used wine instead of tranquilizers. Not only did it help the patients sleep, it also improved their morale and overall satisfaction.[5] In other words, alcohol helped to relieve stress in people who were facing a variety of illnesses, were often away from home, and may have been facing financial difficulties as well.

Like a good many studies, a review study published in a 1985 edition of *Drug and Alcohol Dependence* shows that careful imbibing can have a beneficial effect on the mood and behavior of many people. This review gathered together the results of previously published studies and found that low and/or moderate consumption of alcohol has many beneficial results on human mood. Specifically, it can reduce stress, increase happiness and sociability, reduce tension, lighten depression, ease self-consciousness, boost certain types of cognitive performance, and help with some of the psychiatric problems associated with aging. The author notes that "results from many of the studies reviewed suggest that light or moderate drinking may be beneficial to psychological well-being."[6]

Alcohol can be especially helpful to senior citizens in ill health. Often confined to rest homes or nursing facilities, they may face a special kind of stress exacerbated by their physical ailments, inability to take care of themselves, and loss of control over their daily lives. In 1989, researchers gave hospitalized geriatric patients a little bit of wine or beer every day.[7] The found that the older citizens soon became more social, and were better able to get around on their own.

Simply being more social and regaining some measure of control over life (being able to get around) helps to relieve stress. Researchers at Cushing Hospital had similarly positive results with a group of 34 senile men, only 7 of whom were up and about. When the men were given one bottle of beer a day, they felt livelier. Soon, 25 of them were up and about. Significantly fewer required physical restraint or suffered from incontinence. In another study with senior citizens, one group of senile patients was given beer daily while another group received fruit juice. The ones who drank the beer became more alert and talkative, but the juice drinkers remained quiet and distant. When the beer drinkers were taken off the beverage, or switched to juice, they returned to their previous states.

It's clear that light-to-moderate alcohol consumption can help to keep many people relaxed. Especially when consumed in pleasant company, it can help to lift the mood and relieve stress.

Does it really matter if we're happier? Can feeling a little more like smiling or having a few more pleasant conversations with friends help the majority of people who are *not* ill? The scientific evidence says "yes."

Back in the early 1980s, researchers at the University of Tennessee Health Sciences Center worked with a group of patients suffering from intractable back pain who had not been helped by standard means. The scientists began by measuring the levels of endorphins in the patients' spinal fluid. (Endorphins, the "morphine within" the human body, are hormones that block certain pain signals and help to regulate mood.)

The pain patients were given a placebo ("sugar pill"), but told that they were getting a new medicine that would make them feel better. Soon enough, some 30 percent of them felt better. That's not unusual, for the placebo effect works 30–40 percent of the time. But this is the amazing part. When the doctors rechecked the patients who had improved, they found that their endorphin levels had risen. The increased endorphins were responsible for the pain relief—but what pushed the endorphins up? Not the placebo—that was a worthless sugar pill. It was the patients' thoughts that raised their endorphins. Their positive, anticipatory thoughts actually changed their body chemistry. They didn't simply *think* that they felt better, they really did, and there were changes in body chemistry to prove it.

This phenomenon was confirmed by a group of actors at the University of California. Under the direction of medical researchers, they acted out "happy" and "sad" scenes. When they pretended to be happy, their T-cell proliferative response, a measure of immune system strength, went up. But when they acted sad, it went down. Here was proof that the immune system waxes and wanes with our moods. Being happier and more relaxed makes a positive difference, even if we are already healthy.

IN CONCLUSION

Whether in the form of fear, anger, worry, or depression, stress can be dangerous. In many people, small to moderate amounts of alcohol can help to boost happiness and sociability, while reducing tension, depression, and stress. This means that careful imbibing can help people cope with the demands of life. Of course, there are other ways of dealing with stress, which I'll discuss in Chapter 8, and one should not begin drinking or increase consumption just to handle stress. It's important to know, however, that alcohol can be an antidote to some of the stress-related problems besieging us today.

CHAPTER SEVEN

Drinking, Good Health, and Long Life

SO FAR, WE'VE seen how small to moderate amounts of beer, wine, or spirits can reduce the risk of coronary heart disease, the number-one killer disease in the United States today. The studies showing that conservative imbibing can lower the odds of becoming the victim of an ischemic stroke have also been reviewed, as well as those looking at alcohol's antistress properties. Now let's briefly examine the relationships between alcohol and several other diseases, plus alcohol and aging. Then we'll gather all of the information together to answer what is perhaps the most important question of all: Can drinking extend our lives?

DOES ALCOHOL RAISE BLOOD PRESSURE?

Are those who drink likely to develop high blood pressure (hypertension)? This is an important question, for as I pointed out in previous chapters, elevated blood pressure paves the way for heart disease, stroke, and other ailments. No one doubts that *heavy* drinking raises blood pressure—this has been confirmed by many studies. Along with obesity, heredity, gender, race, and diet, the consumption of more than 30–60 grams of alcohol (3–6 drinks) per day is considered to be a major risk factor for hypertension.[1]

Since it's agreed that *heavy* drinking is deleterious, many people have assumed that light to moderate drinking must also be dangerous.

67

However, some researchers have challenged conventional wisdom, reporting that light to moderate imbibing may not elevate blood pressure. In fact, light drinking may actually *lower* blood pressure in some people. The Munich Blood Pressure Study,[2] the Lubeck Blood Pressure Study,[3] and other research projects have found that in some cases, light drinkers have lower blood pressures than do abstainers. And in the 1977 Kaiser Permanente Study, women who drank 10–20 grams of alcohol per day had lower blood pressures (systolic and diastolic) than did women who consumed no alcohol at all.[4] These findings are certainly not reasons to begin drinking, or to drink more if you already drink, but they do suggest that light to moderate consumption of alcohol may not be the villain it has been made out to be, and may actually be beneficial to some people.

Caution: If you currently have high blood pressure, make sure that you are being treated by a physician and that you discuss all of your habits, including drinking, with him or her. If you suspect that you might have high blood pressure, see your physician immediately.

SHOULD DIABETICS AVOID ALCOHOL?

Diabetes, a major problem in the Western world, is a disease of abundance: There's too much sugar in the bloodstream at certain times. The excess sugar and the upsetting of the body's regulatory mechanisms caused by diabetes damage arteries and increase the risk of heart disease, stroke, kidney failure, blindness, and other serious problems.

In some cases, the diabetic's body is unable to produce enough insulin, the hormone that carries sugar from the bloodstream into the body's cells where it's used for fuel. This kind of diabetes is known as IDDM (insulin dependent diabetes mellitus) or Type I. In the majority of cases, however, diabetics produce normal amounts of insulin, but the body is simply overwhelmed by the harmful effects of poor diet, lack of exercise, and other lifestyle errors. This form of diabetes is referred to as NIDDM (non-insulin dependent diabetes) or Type II.

No one suggests that diabetics should drink heavily, but some researchers have looked into whether or not light drinking could be helpful. Specifically, could alcohol help the body keep the blood sugar under control?

The question was put to the test in 1994 when 40 healthy volunteers were studied at the Stanford University Medical Center.[5] The 20 men and 20 women were classified as either nondrinkers or light-to-moderate (10–30 grams per day) imbibers. To see how their bodies responded to sugar (how well their insulin kept blood sugar under control), they were given large doses of glucose, a kind of sugar. Then samples of their blood were drawn and examined. The light-to-moderate drinkers were better able to keep their blood sugar under control than were the nondrinkers. Even when age, physical activity, body mass index, and the waist-to-hip girth ratio were factored in, it was clear that light-to-moderate drinking helped the body keep blood sugar under control. (It also increased the beneficial HDL cholesterol levels.)

The Stanford study focused on healthy people, leaving open the question as to whether or not alcohol would be helpful to those who already had diabetes. According to a large-scale 1995 study[6] of middle-aged British men, the answer was again yes. The results of this study showed that moderate drinking helped to reduce the risk of developing non-insulin dependent diabetes.

This British study looked at 735 men, ranging in age from 40–59. Compared to "occasional drinkers," the "moderate drinkers" (16–24 units per week) were less likely to develop diabetes.

Although more study is needed, it appears as if alcohol may play a role in helping to keep blood sugar under control, thus assisting in controlling at least one type of diabetes (non-insulin dependent). Light-to-moderate consumption also helps to raise the "good" HDL cholesterol, which can be helpful to diabetics, who are at increased risk of heart disease.

If you have diabetes, don't start drinking or increase your consumption. Instead, ask your doctor what you should do to keep the disease under control.

CAN ALCOHOL AID DIGESTION?

Alcohol has long been considered an aid to digestion and a shield against food-borne bacteria. Before the twentieth century, when water supplies were often contaminated, it was much safer to drink wine, beer, or liquor. No one knew exactly why alcohol was safer to drink back then, but today we know that it has antibacterial properties.

A 1995 study published in the *British Medical Journal*[7] was conducted to see if wine was as effective against "traveler's diarrhea" as bismuth salicylate (the active ingredient in Pepto Bismol and a common remedy for intestinal problems.) Red wine, white wine, tequila, diluted absolute alcohol, bismuth salicylate and sterile water were pitted against "germs" such as salmonella, *Escherichia coli* and shigella. Both wine and bismuth salicylate killed the offending organisms, but the wine did so more effectively.

In addition to destroying certain bacteria, alcohol has other ways of aiding digestion. For example, the sight and smell of alcohol increases salivation in many people. Since saliva contains digestive enzymes, this gets the digestive system rolling.

If you have digestive or gastrointestinal problems, be careful, since heavy drinking can irritate or damage the lining of the stomach. Do not self-medicate by drinking alcohol. Instead, see your physician.

DOES ALCOHOL ENCOURAGE OR PREVENT GALLSTONES?

Technically known as cholelithiasis, gallstones are concentrations of mineral salts and cholesterol found in the gall bladder. They are caused by inability of the gall bladder to properly empty itself, or by obesity, a high-fat and low fiber diet, smoking, genetics, or other factors. Many people with gallstones have no symptoms, while others experience pain, nausea, vomiting, and other problems. *Excessive* drinking is believed to contribute to gallstones, but lesser amounts *may* be helpful.

Twelve healthy volunteers,[8] all light drinkers, were asked to consume 39 grams of alcohol (3–4 drinks) a day for six weeks, then to abstain for another six weeks. While they were drinking, their "good" HDL cholesterol levels rose significantly, and their bile cholesterol saturation indexes fell. This was good news, suggesting that moderate alcohol consumption may be helpful in preventing cholesterol-based gallstones.

But don't start drinking or increase your consumption as a way to prevent or treat gallstones. If you have gallstones or any symptoms of this disease, see your physician.

IS ALCOHOL A CURE FOR THE COMMON COLD?

The cure for the common cold has been sought after as eagerly as the fountain of youth and with about as much success. There is no cure for the cold, but at least one study published in the *American Journal of Public Health*[9] suggests that drinking may help nonsmokers resist this annoying viral infection. Scientists from the Department of Psychology at Carnegie Mellon University deliberately exposed 391 subjects to respiratory viruses. They found that the smokers in the group were more likely than the nonsmokers to develop colds, confirming the common wisdom that smokers get more colds. But this is the interesting part: The nonsmokers who drank up to 3 or 4 alcoholic drinks per day were less likely to come down with a cold than the nonsmokers who did not drink. This one study is not proof, but it suggests that drinking offers nonsmokers a small measure of protection against the common infections that leave us feeling stuffy and miserable.

If you should have serious respiratory problems, however, consult your physician.

DOES ALCOHOL CAUSE CANCER?

The very word "cancer" scares us, and with good reason. Cancer is a deadly disease, and its treatment is often unpleasant and unsuccessful. Cancer is the number-two killer disease in the United States, right behind coronary heart disease, claiming hundreds of thousands of lives every year. We know that many things can cause cancer, including smoking and exposure to asbestos and certain chemicals. The standard American high-fat diet has been implicated in many cancers, including those of the prostate and the breast. We also suspect that genetic susceptibilities play a role in cancer, which would explain why some smokers get cancer while others who puff away for decades do not.

Does alcohol cause cancer? The answer is yes, no, and maybe. According to standard laboratory tests with animals, ethanol is not a carcinogen—it does not cause cancer. When laboratory mice are given drinking fluid that's 43 percent ethanol for up to 2–3 years, they do not develop more tumors than mice who drink regular water.

But even though ethyl alcohol itself does not appear to be a carcinogen, some cancers have been linked to drinking. Ethanol apparently acts as a *cocarcinogen*. A cocarcinogen does not cause cancer by itself, but "strengthens" other potential cancer causers such as cigarette smoke. That's why studies have shown that drinking can increase the risk of developing several types of cancer, including those of the mouth, esophagus, pharynx, and larynx. Many studies have also suggested that cancers of the colon and rectum, and breast cancer in women, are also associated with alcohol consumption.

Where cancer is concerned, it's best to be safe. If you have a family history of cancer, if you smoke, if you consume a high-fat diet, or have any other risk factors for any type of cancer, it's best to abstain from drinking. Completely.

Is It Safe for Senior Citizens to Drink?

Although our elderly population is healthier than ever, some concerned people feel that older bodies are no longer be able to handle alcohol, therefore seniors should not drink. Is this true? Is moderate drinking a problem for those over, say, the age of sixty or sixty-five? The best available evidence suggests that people can continue drinking in moderation well into their sunset years, as long as they don't have health problems that would otherwise make it unwise for them to imbibe. In fact, small amounts of alcohol have been credited with stimulating the appetite and promoting regular bowel function in the elderly, as well as improving their moods while relieving stress and depression.[10]

The body certainly changes as we age, so we can't always apply the results of studies involving young or middle-aged people to the elderly. That's why it is important to repeat certain studies using older subjects. A 1992 study reported in the *Journal of the American Geriatric Society*[11] examined the effects of alcohol on the elderly. This study was designed to "determine whether there is a relationship of low to moderate alcohol consumption with cardiovascular mortality in the elderly." Three groups of men and women, all aged sixty-five or older, were examined. One group was in East Boston, one in New Haven, and the third in Iowa. Those who already had suffered heart attacks, stroke, or cancer were excluded from the study. The results? Data from East Boston and New Haven showed that light-to-moderate alcohol consumption lessened the risk of dying from cardiovascular disease, as well the total risk of dying. (But in Iowa, there was no such improvement.)

There is a downside to drinking for the elderly, of course, just as there is for the young. Alcohol can interfere with sleep and may worsen memory problems, so those with insomnia or existing memory ailments should refrain from drinking. Otherwise, if one is in good physical and mental health, light-to-moderate drinking appears to be safe for senior citizens.

IS ALCOHOL HARMFUL TO THOSE WITH
PSYCHOLOGICAL DISTRESS?

Drinking might worsen certain preexisting psychological conditions. Someone who is depressed, for example, may become even more depressed when drinking. Overall, however, light-to-moderate consumption is not believed to cause any psychological ailments. And there may be some benefit to drinking, at least in certain cases. For some, a glass of beer might be the best medicine.

Beer was compared to thioridazine (a drug used to reduce anxiety and agitation) in an interesting study published in the *New England Journal of Medicine*.[12] The study's subjects were divided into four groups. Instead of taking their regular medicine, Group #1 was given 12 ounces of beer in a pub. Group #2 was given fruit juice in a pub, while Group #3 received thioridazine (their regular medicine) in the pub. Group #4 got thioridazine in the wards (the regular medicine in the regular setting).

The results? The ones who drank beer in the pub showed the most improvement. But wait: Was it the beer that made them feel better, or was it getting out and going to the pub that did the trick? It was the beer, for the group that drank fruit juice in the pub showed almost no improvement at all, and the ones who took their regular medicine in the pub showed only slight improvement. Something in the beer helped these people feel less anxious and agitated.

Of course, alcohol is *not* a substitute for psychological or psychiatric treatment. If you are having any difficulties of this nature, see your physician or psychologist immediately.

DOES ALCOHOL IMPROVE OUR OVERALL HEALTH?

"Overall health" is a difficult concept to describe and analyze. Good health is partially a subjective feeling—some people with recognizable diseases feel fine, while others with no known ailments have pains and other problems. We can assume, however, that people who do not feel well are more likely to go to their doctors' offices and to hospitals. This means that we can look at the way people use health-care facilities as a rough gauge of their feeling of overall health.

Several studies have indeed found that light and moderate drinkers

Alcohol and Prescription Drugs

> ALCOHOL AND MEDICINES are not always a good mix. Alcohol can interact with a medicine, making it less effective or enhancing its side effects. In some cases, the combination of alcohol and medicine can create new and dangerous side effects. Be sure to discuss your drinking habits with your physician or pharmacist before taking any prescription or over-the-counter medications.

use health-care facilities less than do either abstainers or heavy drinkers. This suggests that light-to-moderate imbibers are healthier than those who either refrain from drinking or drink to excess.

The 1983 National Health Interview Survey[13] looked at 17,600 people, comparing their alcohol consumption to their use of acute care facilities in the past twelve months. The participants were classified as current drinkers, past drinkers, or lifelong abstainers. The findings were adjusted to account for age, race, income, and smoking habits, and going to the hospital to deliver a baby was not counted. The results showed that current drinkers are less likely to be hospitalized than lifelong abstainers. In other words, drinking seems to make one healthier, or at least feel healthier. (Best off were the women who had consumed 29–42 alcoholic beverages in the two-week period prior to filling out the study questionnaires, for they were the least likely to go to the hospital.) These results were seconded by a Spanish study,[14] which found that moderate drinkers were less likely than abstainers to use health-care services (specifically hospital and ambulatory care).

But don't start drinking as a way to stay out of the hospital. If you feel that you need medical care, get it immediately.

THE KEY QUESTION:
DOES DRINKING EXTEND OUR LIVES?

Theoretically, conservative consumption of alcoholic beverages should make us live longer, on average. After all, it reduces the risk of coronary heart disease, which is the number-one killer disease in this country today. Half of us fall victim to coronary heart disease. If we can beat heart disease, we should live longer. Alas, theory and reality are not always the same thing. That's why it's necessary to put the theory to the test in rigorous studies. Fortunately, the results of the studies are positive: Light-to-moderate consumption of alcohol extends our lives by reducing the risk of dying.

Let me be clear about one thing: The risk of death due to auto accidents and certain other causes *rises* with alcohol consumption. It's only because the death rate due to coronary heart disease and other problems drops so dramatically that the *overall risk of death* falls among light and moderate imbibers. Of course, everyone eventually dies, no matter how much or how little alcohol is consumed. Light-to-moderate consumption can, however, delay death.

You can clearly see the link between alcohol and longer life in the following chart. Notice that abstainers have a "relative risk" of dying of 1.0. That number is arbitrarily assigned to serve as a reference point. The relative risk drops below 1.0 among light-to-moderate drinkers, indicating that they're likely to live longer than the abstainers. But as the amount of alcohol consumed grows, the relative risk climbs and often goes above 1.0, proving that heavy drinking is not only a health risk, it's downright deadly.

Now let's take a more detailed look at some of the key studies showing that light-to-moderate consumption of alcohol can extend life.

The famous and highly respected Framingham Study[15] found evidence supporting the contention that moderate amounts of alcohol added years to one's life.

STUDY SUMMARY: Drinking habits and the causes and rates of death were studied in 5,209 men and women from Framingham, Massachusetts. RESULTS: This large-scale study found that drinking lowered mortality in men. Specifically, light drinkers among the men had the lowest mortality. The study found no benefit, however, for women who drank.

Relative Risk of Dying of All Causes[16]
According to Level of Reported Usual Alcohol Intake
(adjusted for smoking and other risk factors)

Study	Alcohol Category (number of drinks)	Relative Risk
Japanese Physician's Study[17] This study, published in 1986, followed the participants for 19 years.	None	1.00
	Occasional	0.86
	1–4 per day	0.91
	5+ per day	1.28
	Ex-drinker	1.38
British Regional Heart Study[18] This study, published in 1988, followed the participants for 7.5 years.	Occasional	1.0
	0.1–2 per day	0.7
	2–6 per day	0.7
	6 or more per day	0.9
American Cancer Society[19] This study, published in 1990, followed the participants for 12 years.	Nondrinker	1.00
	Occasional	0.888
	1 per day	0.84
	2 per day	0.93
	3 per day	1.02
	4 per day	1.08
	5 per day	1.22
	6 or more per day	1.38
	Irregular	1.01
Kaiser Pemanente Study[20] The study, published in 1990, followed the participants for less than 7 years.	Abstainers	1.0
	Less than 1 per month	1.0
	1 per month to 1 per day	0.9
	1–2 per day	0.9
	3–5 per day	1.0
	6 or more per day	1.4
	Ex-drinkers	1.1

Study	Alcohol Category (number of drinks)	Relative Risk	
Busselton Study[21] This study, published in 1991, followed the participants for 23 years.	None	1.00	
	Mild	0.92	
	Moderate	0.66	
	Ex-drinkers	1.26	
Kaiser Pemanente Study[22] This study, published in 1992, followed the participants for less than 10 years.		*White*	*Black*
	Abstainers	1.0	1.0
	Less than 1 per month	1.0	0.9
	1 per month to 1 per day	0.8	0.9
	1–2 per day	0.9	0.9
	3–5 per day	1.0	1.1
	6 or more per day	1.2	1.3
	Ex-drinkers	1.3	1.0
British Doctor's Study[23] This study, published in 1991, followed the participants for 12 years.	0	1.00	
	0.1–1.3 per day	0.64	
	1.3–2.7 per day	0.78	
	2.8–4.1 per day	0.72	
	4.2–5.6 per day	0.73	
	5.7 or more per day	1.03	

A 1992 study published in the *Journal of Studies on Alcohol*[24] looked at whether or not consumption of alcoholic beverages reduced the risk of coronary heart disease and added years to life.

STUDY SUMMARY: In 1973, 1,823 men who were free of serious or chronic diseases answered questions about their drinking habits. The men were divided into three age groups and were followed for 12 years. RESULTS: In each age group, the moderate drinkers had the best, meaning the lowest, rates of overall mortality (death).

This study also looked into a second question: Would a moderate drinker live longer even if he had had a drinking problem in the past, or had changed his drinking habits? The answer was yes. The researchers reported that "drinking heavily in the past, ever having tried to quit drinking and having had problems with alcohol were not related to increased risk" of coronary heart disease or death from all causes. In other words, it is possible to overcome *some* of the risks of heavy drinking by reverting to moderate consumption, and to enjoy the protective effects of alcohol once again.

This study presented in *Nutrition Research* in 1991[25] followed a group of people for many years in order to see which lifestyle variables influenced life expectancy.

STUDY SUMMARY: The study was designed to see if the length of one's life could be predicted by measuring factors such as alcohol consumption, energy and fat intake, smoking habits, body mass index, and participation in athletics while in college. A group of White male college graduates, who attended college prior to 1938, filled out lifestyle surveys on five different occasions between 1952 and 1984. RESULTS: The men who drank alcohol lived longer than those who did not. Participation in college athletics or aerobic activities in leisure time, however, did not extend survival time.

The American Cancer Society, an organization that has no reason to champion alcohol, found evidence that alcohol had a positive effect on overall longevity.[26]

STUDY SUMMARY: The study began in 1959, when 276,802 men in the United States, ranging in age from 40–59, were enrolled in a prospective study. During the next 12 years 42,756 of the men died, 18,711 of them from coronary heart disease. The 55.3 percent of the men who were nondrinkers were used as references to develop age and smoking-stratified relative risks of dying (of all causes). RESULTS: Nondrinkers were assigned a relative risk of dying of 1.0. Occasional drinking produced a lesser relative risk of 0.88. The relative risk of dying dropped as low as 0.84 among those who consumed 1 alcoholic beverage per day, then began climbing back up. Even at 6 drinks per day, however, the relative risk of dying of all causes was only 0.92, less than the abstainers' risk of dying.

This report of a ten-year study[27] appearing in a 1981 issue of the British journal *Lancet* confirmed that moderate alcohol consumption helped to add years to life.

STUDY SUMMARY: 1,422 male civil servants were grouped according to the amount of alcohol they consumed daily, and followed for 10 years. RESULTS: Moderate drinkers had lower mortality (death) rates than abstainers and heavy drinkers. There was a U-shaped relationship between alcohol consumption and mortality, with the risk of death dropping as alcohol intake increased from none to light and moderate, then turning up and increasing as intake became heavy. The positive effects of light-to-moderate drinking (and the negative effects of heavy drinking) withstood adjustments for smoking habits, blood pressure, cholesterol levels, and employment grade.

The evidence from each individual study is bolstered by the fact that the findings in the various studies are remarkably consistent even when conducted in different parts of the world, using different ethnic and age groups and both sexes. And it doesn't seem to matter what type of alcoholic beverage one drinks, beer, wine, or distilled spirits, for they all appear to help extend the life span when taken in moderation.[28]

SHOULD ONE DRINK?

The evidence is strong, suggesting that light-to-moderate consumption of alcohol helps to reduce the risk of coronary heart disease and "blockage" stroke, relieve stress, improve other aspects of health, and reduce the overall risk of death. But don't think of alcohol as a cure-all, for even small amounts pose risks for some people, and the dangers of heavy drinking are well known.

Rather than looking upon alcohol as either wonderful or terrible, we should recognize that it, like almost everything else in life, has good points and bad, strengths and weaknesses. The fact that moderate consumption reduces the risk of coronary heart disease is good news for middle-aged men and others at risk for the disease. But it may not be nearly as "medicinal" for a young woman, who already has a relatively low risk of suffering a heart attack, because alcohol can increase her odds of developing breast cancer.

There is no doubt that careful drinking can promote health in many people, and alcohol can fit quite nicely into a healthy lifestyle. Let's take a look at that healthy lifestyle now—and how you can enjoy all the health benefits of alcohol *without* drinking.

CHAPTER EIGHT

Alcohol and the Healthy Lifestyle

IN JANUARY 1996, the United States government acknowledged for the first time ever that light-to-moderate consumption of alcohol could be healthful, and that alcohol had a role to play in a healthy diet and a healthy lifestyle. This represented a major shift in thinking, for up until that time, the government had insisted that alcohol had absolutely no health benefits and should be avoided.

The 1995 "Dietary Guidelines For Americans," issued jointly by the United States Department of Agriculture and the Department of Health and Human Services in January 1996, proclaimed that "Current evidence suggests that moderate drinking is associated with a lower risk of coronary heart disease in some individuals."[1] When the "Guidelines" were made public, assistant secretary of Health Dr. Philip Lee added: "There was a significant bias in the past against drinking. To move from anti-alcohol to health benefits is a big step."[2]

Many studies testifying to the health benefits of light-to-moderate alcohol consumption have been published in major medical journals, including the *Journal of the American Medical Association, Lancet, Annals of Internal Medicine,* the *American Journal of Epidemiology,* the *American Journal of Cardiology*, and the *British Medical Journal*. These studies are part of the wealth of scientific evidence that suggests that small-to-moderate amounts of alcohol may help to:

- reduce the risk of heart disease and stroke by raising the protective HDL cholesterol
- reduce the risk of heart disease and stroke by "thinning" the blood, which makes it less likely that dangerous clots will form and then lodge in heart or brain arteries

- ameliorate some of the harmful effects of stress
- keep blood sugar under control
- protect against gallstones
- lessen the need for medical care overall
- reduce the relative risk of dying from all causes by 10–30 percent

But remember, a good diet and moderate use of alcohol are only two of the many tools we can use to build good health. Exercise, a positive outlook on life, and other healthy lifestyle habits can also add years to your life—and life to your years. That's why we should use as many health tools as possible, making sure not to neglect any of them.

With that in mind, let's take a look at the "Dietary Guidelines For Americans" and then at some other ways of getting and staying healthy.

"Dietary Guidelines for Americans"

There's much more to the food we eat than vitamins, minerals, and calories. The right foods also have "medicinal" effects, helping to strengthen our immune systems and protect us from a variety of major and minor ailments. According to Donna Shalala, secretary of the Department of Health and Human Services, "For most Americans who do not smoke or engage in substance abuse, a good, balanced diet is the most important thing we can do for ourselves to promote health and long life. A good diet reduces the risk of premature death from our biggest killers—including heart disease, some cancers, stroke, and diabetes."[3]

Here are the seven components of a healthy lifestyle, as described by the United States government health officials:

1) Eat a variety of foods

The body needs plentiful amounts of a variety of vitamins and minerals on a daily basis. It also needs a number of phytochemicals (special substances found in plants) such as lycopene, quercetin, and resveratrol that promote health. Some phytochemicals act as natural blood thinners. Others have antibiotic or anti-inflammatory properties. Still others function as antioxidants to help the body fight off cancer and heart disease.

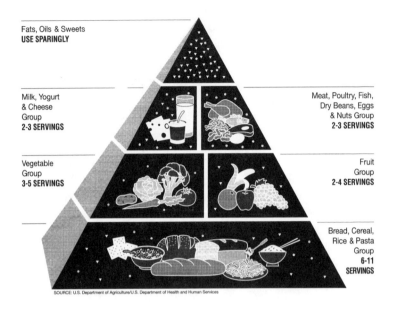

Fats, Oils & Sweets
USE SPARINGLY

Milk, Yogurt
& Cheese
Group
2-3 SERVINGS

Meat, Poultry, Fish,
Dry Beans, Eggs
& Nuts Group
2-3 SERVINGS

Vegetable
Group
3-5 SERVINGS

Fruit
Group
2-4 SERVINGS

Bread, Cereal,
Rice & Pasta
Group
**6-11
SERVINGS**

SOURCE: U.S. Department of Agriculture/U.S. Department of Health and Human Services

Consuming a variety of foods is the best way of making sure that you get all of the many nutrients your body needs. Protein, carbohydrates, fats, vitamins, minerals, and phytochemicals are found in different amounts and different combinations in various foods. Since no single food contains enough of everything, you'll miss out on important building blocks for good health if you eat the same few foods over and over again. Eating a variety of foods is also important because the nutrients in one food can help the body absorb substances from another.

How do you know whether you're eating enough (or too much) of any one food? Use the Food Guide Pyramid to help you make intelligent choices.

Let's take a closer look at the pyramid:

- *Bread, Cereal, Rice, and Pasta*—6–11 servings—For optimal health, a good portion of your diet should be made up of bread, cereal, rice, and pasta. Six to eleven servings from this group every day may sound like a lot, but remember that just one slice of bread, one ounce of cereal, or ½ cup of pasta counts as a full serving. If you have an ounce of cereal and a piece of toast at breakfast, a sandwich for lunch, and a cup of pasta at dinner, you'll get your six servings. But remember to be imaginative. Instead of limiting yourself to just bread, white rice, and spaghetti, (the standard selections), try barley, buckwheat, millet, oats, rye, and "short" and "long" whole grain rice.

- *Vegetables*—3–5 servings—How much is a serving? The rule of thumb is that one serving equals one cup of the vegetable raw, ½ cup cooked, or ¾ cup of vegetable juice. There are a number of vegetables to choose from in the typical supermarket, including artichokes, asparagus, beet greens, beets, broccoli, Brussels sprouts, red cabbage, green cabbage, Chinese cabbage, carrots, cauliflower, celery, cucumbers, eggplant, garlic, ginger, jicama, leeks, many types of lettuce and mushrooms, green peppers, red peppers, yellow peppers, okra, onions, parsley, potatoes, radishes, spinach, and a wide variety of squashes. Because they come from the ground, not from animals, vegetables contain absolutely no cholesterol. They tend to be low in fat, sugar, and sodium, with good amounts of fiber, complex carbohydrates, vitamins, minerals, phytochemicals, and enzymes. Be sure to vary your selection rather than eat the same two or three again and again. And it's best to eat vegetables lightly cooked, for overcooking can damage some of their nutrients. Some vegetables, such as carrots, cucumbers, celery, broccoli, and cauliflower make great "finger foods." They're highly nutritious when served fresh and uncooked, for their nutrients haven't been damaged or destroyed by cooking or processing. *A final note:* If you drink vegetable juice, be sure to count the juice toward no more than one of your vegetable servings per day. Vegetable juice is nutritious but it contains very little fiber, which is an important part of the diet.
- *Fruit*—2–4 servings—One serving of fruit equals either one medium fruit (such as an apple, banana, or orange), ½ cup of a chopped, cooked, or canned fruit, or ¾ cup fruit juice. You can choose from a tremendous amount of fruits, including apples, apricots, bananas, several kinds of berries, cantaloupes, cherries, figs, grapes, guavas, mangoes, oranges, papayas, peaches, pears, persimmons, pineapples, plums, pomegranates, tomatoes, and watermelon. (Yes, the tomato is technically a fruit, not a vegetable.) Generally low in fat and sodium, with absolutely no cholesterol, fruits offer nutrition mixed with sweetness. Fresh fruit is the best

choice because its nutrients have not been damaged by heating, canning, drying, or other forms of processing.

Bread, cereal, rice, pasta, vegetables, and fruit should make up the bulk of your diet. If you add up all the recommended servings listed in the Food Guide Pyramid, you'll see that well over 70 percent of your daily intake should come from these groups.

- *Meat, Poultry, Fish, Dried Beans, Eggs, and Nuts*—2–3 servings— Although many of us were raised with the notion that we need large quantities of meat and other "protein" foods to stay healthy, smaller amounts are more than adequate for good health. That's why the government recommends only 2–3 servings from this group daily. A serving size is 2–3 ounces of lean cooked meat, poultry, or fish, or ½ cup of cooked dried beans, peas, or lentils, or 1 egg, or 2 tablespoons of peanut butter. Meat, nuts, and eggs are certainly nutritious, but don't forget that they are also high in fat. Fish, on the other hand, has been linked to heart health. Be adventurous when eating fish! Try abalone, brook trout, cod, flounder, haddock, halibut, red snapper, scallops, sea bass, sole, tuna, yellow perch, and others. And don't forget the omega-3 fatty acids found in salmon, herring, mackerel, and other "deep sea" fish. The omega-3s are believed to protect against heart disease and stroke by helping to keep the blood "thin," thus preventing the formation of unnecessary blood clots that can trigger a heart attack or stroke by lodging in heart or brain arteries.
- *Milk, Yogurt, and Cheese*—2–3 servings—Either 1 cup of milk or yogurt, 1½ ounces of natural cheese, or 2 ounces of processed cheese is considered one serving. This group is an important source of calcium and other nutrients necessary for strong bones.
- *Fats, Oils, and Sweets*—Use sparingly. These foods are usually low in nutrients but high in calories. It's easy to fill up on fat, oils, and sweets, leaving no room in your stomach for the more nutritious foods that you need.

Although the Food Guide Pyramid includes meat, vegetarians can also enjoy balanced, healthful diets by following the government recommendations. This is especially true if they are lacto-ovo-vegetarians who eat the dairy products and eggs that provide the body with much-needed calcium, protein and vitamin B_{12}. But even those who don't eat any animal products can successfully follow the Food Pyramid plan. Dried beans, nuts, or tofu are acceptable substitutes from the Meat Group, and the calcium provided by the Milk, Yogurt, and Cheese Group can be found in canned salmon or sardines (only if you eat their soft bones!), green leafy vegetables (such as bok choy or mustard greens), tofu processed with calcium sulfate, and tortillas made from lime-processed corn. Remember, though, that if you are a strict vegan (no eggs or dairy products), you will need to take a B_{12} supplement, for this vitamin is only found in animal products. It's also difficult to get the required amounts of calcium if you eat no dairy products and iron or zinc if you eat no meat products. Supplementation may then be necessary.

2) BALANCE THE FOOD YOU EAT WITH PHYSICAL ACTIVITY IN ORDER TO MAINTAIN OR IMPROVE YOUR WEIGHT

Being overweight is a little like coming down with a load of viral germs." Excess body fat is not a bacteria or virus, but it does increase the risk of heart disease, stroke, high blood pressure, arthritis, diabetes, some kinds of cancer and other ailments.

Unfortunately, growing numbers of Americans are obese, and children and teenagers are packing on the pounds earlier in life than ever before. Plus the older we get, the more weight we tend to gain as we become more sedentary and our metabolisms slow down. That's why it's important to get into the exercise habit early and to exercise regularly throughout life.

Exercise increases the basal metabolic rate (the rate at which we burn calories), meaning that we'll burn more calories even when we're at rest. Over time, regular walking, jogging, bicycling, rowing, or other aerobic exercises (anything that gets your heart pumping faster and your breath coming harder) can step up your metabolic rate—if you do aerobic exercise for some thirty minutes per session, at least three times a week.

As for maintaining your present weight, just follow this simple formula: Take in the same amount of calories that you burn each day! To gain weight, take in more calories; to lose weight, take in less. Sounds easy, right? But it isn't for many people.

To help control your weight, remember this: If you consistently use just 100 calories more than you take in each day (about what you'd burn on an exercise bike in 15 minutes), you will lose close to a pound a month, or 12 pounds per year. But if you consistently *take in* 100 calories more than you burn each day (the equivalent of two sandwich cookies), you will *gain* nearly a pound a month, or 12 pounds per year! Every calorie in or out is important, so look for small ways to add exercise to your daily routine while lowering your calorie intake. Take the stairs instead of the elevator; park a little further away from the store than you normally do; take a short walk at the end of the day; join a dance class. At the same time, opt for nonfat dairy products and salad dressings; trim the fat off of your meat, poultry, or fish; broil rather than fry; and have fresh fruit rather than layer cake for dessert. These little changes can add up to a big difference in both your weight and your overall health.

Although the average American tends to carry too much weight, too little weight can also be a problem. Becoming overly thin due to strenuous dieting or unhealthy practices such as binging and purging, abnormal use of laxatives or excessive exercising can severely deplete the body of nutrients and may be a sign of deep-rooted psychological problems. Unexplained, sudden weight loss can indicate illness or other health problems. If you're seriously underweight or have suffered an unexplained weight loss, see your physician immediately.

3) CHOOSE A DIET WITH PLENTY OF GRAIN PRODUCTS, VEGETABLES, AND FRUITS

Over 70 percent of a healthful diet consists of grains, fruits, and vegetables. Besides providing complex carbohydrates, vitamins, minerals, and fiber, these foods contain no cholesterol and are associated with lower incidences of many diseases, especially cancer and heart disease.

Fruits and vegetables are excellent sources of many vitamins and minerals, and they usually contain little to no fat (although avocados and a few others are high in fat). Beta carotene and vitamin C (well-known antioxidants that scientists believe can slow the development of cancer and certain other diseases) are found primarily in fruits and vegetables. Fruits and vegetables also provide folic acid, which is essential for healthy fetal development. Many studies have shown that most Americans don't eat enough fruits or vegetables. To get more

Some Tips for Staying Slim

- Eat 5–6 small meals per day, rather than 3 large ones.
- Work little exercise periods into your day: take the stairs whenever possible; park your car at the far end of the parking lot; take a stroll at lunch, et cetera.
- Eat plenty of grains and vegetables. They're low in fat but give you a comfortable feeling of fullness.
- Trim all visible fat off your meat and poultry. And watch out for hidden fats: A single tablespoon of some salad dressings may contain 100 calories.
- Eat slowly. It takes about 20 minutes for satiety (the feeling of being full) to set in, so if you eat slowly, you'll stop sooner. Gobblers eat more.
- Don't eat alone. You'll enjoy your meals more and eat more slowly if you can converse with a good companion.
- Drink at least 8 glasses of water every day. Believe it or not, this helps to prevent water retention (bloating).
- Take advantage of the many delicious nonfat and low-fat products available, including salad dressings, dairy products and, frozen dinners. But watch the calorie count and don't over-do it. Even low-calorie foods can pack on the pounds if you eat too many of them.
- Don't read or watch television while eating. You can down an entire carton of ice cream without knowing it if your attention is focused elsewhere. Pay attention to your food and to the act of eating.

into your diet, begin your meal with a fresh salad that includes vegetables, eat fresh fruit as a snack or dessert, and try more vegetarian dishes.

Grains (bread, pasta, cereals, and rice) are good sources of the complex carbohydrates that provide the body with energy. They also supply B vitamins, minerals, and fiber, and can help you to eat less by giving you a nice, full feeling in the stomach. The fiber found in grains, fruits, and vegetables is particularly important to good health. It comes in two forms—*insoluble fiber* (Grandma used to call it *roughage*), which is primarily found in the bran portion of grains and in most parts of any plant, and *soluble fiber,* which is found in oat bran and pectin. Insoluble fiber helps to speed food through the digestive tract, preventing prolonged contact between potential carcinogens and the lining of the intestines. Soluble fiber helps to soak up excess cholesterol and cancer-promoting bile acids, and then sweep them out of the body. Eating plenty of fiber-containing foods helps to maintain proper functioning of the bowels, control or eliminate constipation, diverticulitis, and hemorrhoids, lower the risk of certain cancers (such as colon cancer) and protect against heart disease. To get more fiber into your diet, eat high-fiber fruits and vegetables (with skins whenever possible) such as carrots, berries, potatoes, peas, corn, or pears. Other high-fiber choices include cooked dried beans, peas, and lentils, and whole grain products.

Grains, vegetables, and fruits are also good sources of phytochemicals. Phytochemicals are nonvitamin, nonmineral substances found in edible plants ("phyto" means plant). Although scientists have only recently begun to understand their tremendous utility in helping the body stay healthy, some predict that in the near future we'll have recommended daily allowances of these powerful health helpers. Here are some of the phytochemicals you'll find in grains, vegetables, and fruits:

- *Ajoene*—a strong blood thinner found in garlic
- *Allicin*—a natural antibiotic found in garlic
- *Alpha-linolenic acid*—an omega-3 fatty acid found in olive oil, canola oil, and other foods that may help to guard against cancer and heart disease
- *Bioflavonoids*—found in the outer layer, skin, and peels of vegetables and fruits, as well as in coffee, tea, wine, and green leafy vegetables
- *Capsaicin*—a "hot" substance with anti-inflammatory properties found in chili peppers that may help the body fight off respiratory ailments and guard against ulcers of the stomach
- *Chlorophyll*—an antioxidant in many vegetables that may protect against cancer
- *Coumarins*—natural blood thinners found in fresh vegetables, fruits, and cereal grains

88

- *Glutathione*—an antioxidant found in watermelon, strawberries, tomatoes, and other foods
- *Indoles*—anticancer compounds found in cabbage, broccoli, Brussels sprouts, and other members of the "crucifer" family of vegetables
- *Lycopene*—an antioxidant found in tomatoes, watermelon, and other foods
- *Phenols*—antiviral substances found in fruits, potatoes, garlic, green tea, and some nuts
- *Quercetin*—a bioflavonoid and naturally occurring antioxidant found in red grapes, red and yellow onions, broccoli, and other foods
- *Terpenes*—cancer-fighting substances found in lemons and other foods

Variety may or may not be the spice of life, but it is certainly the best approach when choosing which fruits, vegetables, and whole grains to eat.

1) CHOOSE A DIET LOW IN FAT, SATURATED FAT, AND CHOLESTEROL

The body needs a small amount of fat to maintain good health, as the fat we eat supplies us with essential fatty acids and fat-soluble vitamins, while the fat we carry on our frames helps to insulate the body and protect vital organs. But too much fat in the diet can lead to obesity, heart disease, stroke, cancer, and diabetes. That's why it's important to keep dietary fat to a safe minimum.

Fat should account for no more than 30 percent of the daily calorie intake. (Calories come in the form of fat, protein, and carbohydrates.) If you're eating 2,000 calories a day, for example, no more than 600 of those calories should come from fat.

Here's another way to look at it. Again, suppose you take in 2,000 calories per day, and that you limit yourself to 600 calories from fat. Since each gram of fat is worth 9 calories, those 600 fat calories equal 65 grams of fat. If you read the labels on packaged foods and consult charts to see how many grams of fat are in fresh foods, you'll be able to keep track of those 65 daily grams of fat. (Take a close look at the food labels. You might be surprised to see that a McDonald's biscuit with sausage and eggs has nearly 40 grams of fat—two-thirds of your

Selected Sources of Some Key Nutrients

Beta carotene (which your body can convert into vitamin A)—apricots, broccoli, cantaloupe, carrots, kale, mangoes, nectarines, papaya, parsley, red chili peppers, spinach, sweet potatoes

Folic acid—apricots, asparagus, beans, broccoli, Brussels sprouts, cantaloupe, carrots, cauliflower, okra, pecans, brown rice, spinach, turnip greens, walnuts

Calcium—almonds, asparagus, barley, green beans, cantaloupe, celery, cherry, garlic, grapes, lemons, low-fat milk, onions, oranges, pineapples, spinach, strawberries, walnuts, water cress

Iron—apricots, navy beans, grapes, lentils, millet, oysters, parsley, peaches, plums, potatoes, sesame seeds, spinach, leafy green vegetables, walnuts, wheat, whole grain oats

Magnesium—apples, bananas, barley, broccoli, cabbage, carrots, corn, garlic, grapes, milk, mushrooms, onions, oranges, parsley, pecans, pineapple, plums, spinach, tomatoes

Potassium—bananas, carrots, flounder, lentils, peaches, potatoes, winter squash, tomatoes, leafy green vegetables

Vitamin A—beef liver, low-fat cheese, milk products

Vitamin B$_1$ (thiamin)—almonds, buckwheat, garlic, lentils, lima beans, millet, navy beans, pinto beans, red beans, whole grain oats, rice, rye, wheat

Vitamin B$_2$ (riboflavin)—almonds, brewer's yeast, broccoli, chicken, lentils, mushrooms, navy beans, okra, parsley, pinto beans, salmon, turkey, wheat bran and germ, wild rice, yogurt

Vitamin B$_3$ (niacin)—almonds, barley, brook trout, buckwheat, chicken, dates, haddock, halibut, prunes, salmon, sesame seeds, split peas, turkey, whole grain rice, wheat

continued

Vitamin B₅ (pantothenic acid)—beans, fish, lentils, nuts, peas, leafy green vegetables, wheat bran and germ, whole grain cereals

Vitamin B₆ (pyridoxine)—albacore, bananas, barley, Brussels sprouts, red cabbage, cantaloupe, cauliflower, garbanzo beans, lentils, navy beans, pinto beans, potatoes, salmon, spinach

Vitamin B₁₂ (cobalamin)—cheese, eggs, haddock, milk, perch, salmon, tuna, yogurt

Vitamin C (ascorbic acid)—asparagus, broccoli, Brussels sprouts, cabbage, cantaloupe, cauliflower, cranberries, grapefruit, guava, lemons, mangoes, okra, oranges, papaya, parsley, raspberries, spinach

Vitamin E (tocopherol)—broccoli, Brussels sprouts, green beans, nuts, milk, peas, tomatoes, leafy green vegetables

Zinc—almonds, black pepper, buckwheat, carrots, chicken, chili powder, corn, haddock, milk, oysters, paprika, sardines, thyme, tuna, whole grain oats and wheat

daily allotment! An Extra Crispy chicken thigh from Kentucky Fried Chicken contains 23 grams of fat. Onion rings from Jack in the Box also have a whopping 23 grams of fat! A single ounce of chocolate covered peanuts contains more than 11 grams of fat. It's no wonder that some people are unknowingly gulping down well over 100 grams of fat per day!)

Here are a few tips to help you lower the amount of fat in your diet:

- eat nonfat or low-fat dairy products (milk, cheese, yogurt, sour cream) instead of the standard versions
- purchase lean or extra-lean meat
- cut all visible fat away from meat or poultry before cooking
- take the skin off of poultry before cooking
- limit the amount of added fats (oil, butter, margarine, salad dressing) to 1 tablespoon (or about 100 calories) per day
- avoid cream soups, gravies, and rich desserts. Use sauces based on nonfat ingredients instead of sauces made with cream, butter or mayonnaise
- rather than standard high-fat salad dressings (and most are fairly

high in fat), flavor your salad with lemon juice, fat-free or low-fat dressing
- eat clear soups made with fat-skimmed broth
- have fresh fruit rather than cake, pie, or ice cream for dessert or snacks
- rely on low-fat grains such as rice or bulgur wheat to fill you up
- avoid salami, sausages, and other processed meats, for they tend to be high in fat

In addition to lowering the amount of fat you take in daily, it's important to pay attention to the kind of fat you're consuming. Fat comes in three forms—saturated, monounsaturated, and polyunsaturated. Saturated fats (the kind found in prime rib, bacon, doughnuts, lard, certain kinds of cake icing and deep fat-fried foods) can clog your arteries and quickly push your cholesterol level up, so keep your saturated fat intake down to no more than 10 percent of your daily calories. If you're eating a 2,000 calorie per day diet, only 600 of those calories should come from fat, and only 200 calories (or 22 grams) from saturated fat.

Finally, choose foods that are low in cholesterol. There are two sources of cholesterol—cholesterol from foods (*dietary cholesterol*) and cholesterol made by the body (*endogenous cholesterol*). Your body makes all the cholesterol you need, using it to build cell walls and construct hormones, among other things. The body tries to compensate for the cholesterol you eat by making less of its own, but a diet high in cholesterol or saturated fat can push your blood cholesterol to dangerously high levels, increasing the risk of heart disease and stroke.

Your daily intake of cholesterol should be restricted to 300 milligrams. Limit the cholesterol-containing foods that you eat and cut back on the foods containing saturated fat, which can also raise blood cholesterol levels. Dietary cholesterol is only found in foods that come from animals, such as egg yolks, meat, organ meats, shellfish, poultry, and fatty milk products. There is absolutely no cholesterol in vegetables, fruits, grains, and other foods that grow below, on, or above the ground.

5) CHOOSE A DIET MODERATE IN SUGARS

Blamed for everything from hyperactivity to diabetes to the blues, sugar has developed quite a black eye in recent years. Most of the charges against the sweetener have not been proven, but that doesn't mean that excess sugar is necessarily *good* for you. Sugar can cause tooth decay and contribute to overweight. Eating sugary foods may also mean that you'll fill up with nutritionally poor foods, leaving no room for the nutritious foods your body needs. Therefore, sugars should be used in moderation—or better yet, sparingly.

Watch out for the hidden sugars in food. When reading labels on packaged food, look for the words "sugar," "brown sugar," "invert sugar," "raw sugar," "dextrose," "maltose," "corn sweetener," "corn syrup," "high-fructose corn syrup," "honey," and "fructose." These are all other names for sugar. If sugar or one of the "code words" for sugar is the first or second ingredient, or if you see several of these code names on the ingredient list, the food is probably loaded with sugar and is best left on the shelf.

6) Choose a Diet Moderate in Salt and Sodium

Medical researchers have also found that salt (sodium) can push up blood pressure in salt-sensitive individuals, and that cultural groups that eat a lot of salt tend to have higher blood pressures than groups that consume less. Since it's impossible to tell in advance who will eventually be affected by a high-salt diet, it's prudent for all of us to watch our salt intakes.

One thing is clear: Most of us consume a lot more salt than actually we need (about one teaspoon daily). Since too much salt is potentially harmful, it's wise to find ways to cut back. Many people find that after they've lowered their sodium intakes for a while, their taste for salt weakens and they can't consume as much as they once did. To cut back on sodium and salt, consider the following:

- add less salt to your food at the table (or throw away the saltshaker altogether)
- add less salt than the recipe calls for when cooking
- avoid processed, frozen, or pickled foods, which tend to have lots of added salt
- use low-sodium products
- cut back on salty condiments such as soy sauce, BBQ sauce, and salad dressings
- avoid chips, pretzels, salted nuts, and other salty snacks

- eat plenty of fresh fruits, vegetables, and whole grains, which are naturally low in salt

7) If You Drink Alcoholic Beverages, Do So in Moderation

For the first time ever, the United States government has recently recognized that alcohol can be a tasty and healthful addition to the diet. Light-to-moderate consumption of alcohol has been shown to decrease the risk of heart disease and otherwise promote health in some people. Still, it's important to remember that alcoholic beverages supply calories but few nutrients. Like sugary foods, alcoholic beverages can fill you up, leaving no room for the necessary nutritious foods.

Beware of excessive intake, for it is associated with increased heart disease, stroke, cancer, birth defects, and overall violence. If you drink, do so in moderation.

Certain people should not drink, including children and adolescents, pregnant women or those trying to conceive, anyone who is planning to drive or do anything that requires skill, those taking medications, and those who have trouble restricting their drinking. It is recommended that all drinking take place in conjunction with meals, in moderation, and only when doing so will not put anyone at risk.

Beating "Thought Disease"

Following the U.S. Government's "Dietary Guidelines For Americans" can help you to live young and healthy, full of energy, to a very old age. But diet and exercise are only the beginning. We can strengthen our health even more by applying the lessons learned by a new branch of medical science called psychoneuroimmunology, the study of the mind-body connection. Studies pouring in from laboratories across the country and in Europe are showing that our thoughts have a profound influence on our physical health, and that we can use the mind-body connection to increase our resistance to many diseases.

When I was a young boy, I accompanied my physician-father to the hospital late one night. He had been called to examine an elderly woman who had been in a deep coma for three days. The neurosurgeon, who was going to perform exploratory brain surgery the next

"The Dietary Guidelines For Americans," Summarized

- eat a variety of foods
- balance the food you eat with physical activity to maintain or improve your weight
- choose a diet with plenty of grain products, vegetables, and fruits
- choose a diet low in fat, saturated fat, and cholesterol
- choose a diet moderate in sugars
- choose a diet moderate in salt and sodium
- if you drink alcoholic beverages, do so in moderation

(To learn more about healthful eating, read the books listed in the "Eating For Health" section of the Bibliography.)

morning, wanted my father to make sure that the woman was strong enough to withstand the surgery.

Immediately upon arriving at the hospital, my father and I were directed to the proper room by a nurse. We walked rapidly down the darkened hallway, the nurse following slowly behind, and pushed open the very heavy door to the patient's room to see a woman lying flat on her back in bed, looking stiff as a board. Needles and tubes were stuck into various parts of her body.

On an impulse, my father put his mouth right up next to her ear and shouted "WAKE UP!" I nearly jumped out of my skin as her eyes flew open and she bolted up in bed, wide awake. Before anyone could say anything, the nurse pushed open the door and, seeing that the woman was awake, shouted "You cured her, you cured her! It's a miracle!" Then she ran off to tell the other nurses about this miraculous cure.

We later learned that the elderly, nearly deaf woman had become dizzy at home, so she lay down in bed. Her daughter walked in and, thinking that her mother had passed out (or worse), called for help. Soon the woman found herself surrounded by emergency personnel who shouted at her, shined lights in her face, and pushed needles into her arms and legs. Confused and frightened, the poor woman suffered a reaction in which her mental distress was converted into the physical symptoms of a coma. The more they did to her in her home and at the hospital, the more frightened she became. So she lay in the coma-like state until someone came along and told her to "Wake up!"

Most of us are not in a coma, but neither are we fully awake and living life. We're sometimes a little frightened and confused by events, we feel helpless to make things better, we worry about losing our jobs or loved ones, we fear we'll fail the next test or review. Unfortunately, our distress does not remain in our heads.

You see, there is never a thought without a corresponding "thing" in the body. Every thought we think has some effect on the body. Good thoughts produce good "things," such as the endorphin hormones that block pain, elevate the mood, and possibly even work with the immune system to defeat some diseases. But "bad" thoughts, such as the fear that triggers the "fight or flight" response, invariably lead to an increase of high-voltage chemicals in the body that can weaken the immune system. Many doctors have suspected that unhappy thoughts weaken the body, but this notion couldn't be proven until the early 1970s, when researchers found nerve connections linking the brain and the nervous system to the bone marrow, thymus, spleen, lymph tissue, and other immune system "staging areas." These findings proved that while the mind/nervous system might not communicate directly with the individual immune system cells, they sure seemed to "talk" to the places where the immune "soldiers" grew up, where they were trained, and where they "went to work."

Unfortunately, many of our minds have become so filled with negative thoughts as opportunities have passed us by, as relationships have failed, as dreams have faded. Optimism and enthusiasm for life have been replaced by thoughts of "I can't," "It won't work," "I'm not good enough," "Why bother?" and "Why me? God, why me?" With negative thoughts filling our minds and negative "things" affecting our bodies, many of us are suffering from "thought disease." The effects of "thought disease" are widespread. It can fill the body with high-voltage chemicals that shock the heart, constrict the arteries, encourage potentially deadly blood clotting, and weaken the immune system.

It's "thought disease" that killed the frightened rocket scientists and laboratory animals described in Chapter 4. It's "thought disease" that pushes up cholesterol in accountants during the stress-filled tax season every year. And it's "thought disease" that made West Point cadets more susceptible to infectious mononucleosis. Expected to be the best, mentally and physically, at all times, West Point cadets are under a lot of stress. The "thought disease"/stress/illness connection was examined when slightly over 1,300 West Point cadets had their blood tested for the Epstein-Barr virus antibody (EBV). The presence of EBV is an indicator of infectious mononucleosis. Only those cadets who did not have the EBV antibody were followed. (Those who already had the antibodies were eliminated from the study.)

Some of the cadets undergoing the rigorous physical and mental training remained healthy, while others became positive for EBV, and still others developed mono. The cadets who actually developed mono reported feeling more pressure, and had poor academic performances. In other words, the ones who felt the most stressed got sick! They were all eating the same food, going to the same classes, doing the same exercises. The big difference was how they felt about what was happening, and that difference in their stressful thoughts resulted in an increased susceptibility to mono.

It's not just future army officers whose immune systems can suffer from stress. Imagine being an astronaut up in space. At the end of your journey you find yourself hurtling toward Earth, hoping the ship will not burn up during reentry and that the parachute will open! During the first four days after splashdown, a markedly stressful event, our Skylab astronauts suffered from a reduced T-cell response. (T cells are important immune system soldiers. With weakened T cells, the immune system is not at full strength.)

We've also learned that losing a beloved spouse leads to a decrease in the ability of the survivor to respond to challenges (such as "germs") as long as eight weeks later. Other studies have shown that immune systems are thrown for a loop when people are taking care of severely ill loved ones, when they are going through difficult divorces, and when they are preparing for or taking important tests. Granted, losing a spouse, being a West Point cadet, or blasting off into outer space are extremely stressful situations that we don't face every day. But they serve as examples of what can happen when unhappy thoughts become unhappy "things" within the body.

Other studies illustrate what can happen when happy thoughts within our heads are converted to health-enhancing "things" within the body. For example, the endorphin/back pain study described in Chapter 6 shows how hopeful anticipation can increase the supply of endorphins within the body. And the actor's study described in the same chapter points to the link between "happy" thoughts and the strengthening of the immune system.

In a fascinating look at the power of thoughts, researchers found that positive, anticipatory thoughts could even help to stave off death, at least temporarily. They noted that mortality among Jewish men dropped significantly shortly before the important holiday of Passover. After Passover, the death rate leapt above normal, high enough to compensate for the earlier drop in the deaths before Passover. Then the death rate settled back to normal. The researchers concluded that the joyful anticipation of Passover helped to strengthen some Jewish men enough to keep them alive through the holiday. Researchers at the University of California confirmed this finding by examining the death rates among elderly Chinese women before, during, and after the Harvest Moon Festival (which places great emphasis on the symbolic importance of elderly women). Somehow, the happy anticipation of the holiday kept them alive a little longer.

The bad news is that "thought disease" begins with our thoughts. But that's also the good news, for we have absolute control over our thoughts. We can choose the positive thoughts that helped the pain patients increase their endorphin levels, strengthened the actors' immune systems, and gave the Jewish men and Chinese women the strength to lengthen their lives. This is nothing new, although our ability to prove that mind and body are connected is a recent development. The Bible, ancient Roman and Greek philosophers, and other scholars throughout the ages have noted that people who dwell on the hurts they have suffered tend to be sicker than those whose minds are filled with thoughts of joy, love, and beauty. We, as individuals, are the only ones who put thoughts into our heads. This means that we can choose to focus on the positive, letting those thoughts become positive and healthful "things" within our bodies.

Lifestyle Habits of the Healthy

As the baby boomers enter middle age, there is increased interest in finding the fountain of youth that will keep us young in mind and body well into our seventies and eighties (if not longer!). A growing number of medical researchers are investigating melatonin, deprenyl, Gerovital, DHEA (dehydroepiandrosterone), and other substances that may help to extend life. Scientists will undoubtedly perfect some

Reducing Stress—without Alcohol

CONSUMING LIGHT TO moderate amounts of alcohol is only one way of reducing stress. There are many other approaches, including:

• quit racing against the clock. Walk a little slower, talk a little slower, drive in the slow lane. Leave earlier when you're going somewhere so you won't have to worry about getting there on time
• relax, even if only for a short time, every single day
• have fun, even if only for a few minutes, every single day. Visit friends, play a game, watch a funny movie, read an enjoyable book, or do whatever it takes to bring a smile to your lips
• exercise every day. You don't have to break weight-lifting or running records while exercising. If you like, you can simply garden, stroll briskly through the park, or ride a bicycle through the neighborhood. Many people have found that meditation, yoga, and stretching classes help them combat stress
• spend as much time as possible with friends and loved ones. Look upon every birthday, anniversary, holiday, graduation, or other occasion as a chance to enjoy the company of wonderful people
• rather than allowing yourself to become isolated, make yourself a vital and active part of your family and community. Meet your neighbors, join a club or church or civic organization, do volunteer work for a local charity, take a class at the nearby community college or adult education center
• don't try to be all things to all people. Don't try to solve everyone's problems, every time. Help when you can, but don't run yourself into the ground trying to do for others. That hurts both you and them
• don't plan to do more than you can comfortably handle in any given day

continued

- act, walk, and talk as if you were enthusiastic about life. You may not be so sanguine when you begin, but when you act, walk, and talk as if you are, it's likely that you will be soon
- look upon every problem as a new opportunity to excel
- if you don't believe in yourself, pretend that you do. Behaving as if you believe in yourself is like planting a seed—the real belief will grow, with time
- don't worry about it if you can't finish everything you think you should.
- only a corpse is completely finished

Finally, remember what the great American philosopher Ralph Waldo Emerson said about thoughts: "A man is what he thinks all day long." If you think about stress and unhappiness all day long, you're unwittingly setting the stage for distress. But if you think of joy and success, you're on your way to pushing stress aside.

of the "wonder drugs" in time, but meanwhile, here are a few things we've learned about aging and health. These are simple tips from healthy and active senior citizens, the people who know the most about living young and healthy into old age. Healthy oldsters tend to have some traits and habits in common, including:

- optimism
- serenity
- not smoking
- drinking in moderation
- getting 7–8 hours sleep every night
- eating three regular meals per day, especially breakfast
- exercising regularly
- remaining active and social

It's all very simple. But these simple habits and traits have been associated with health and longevity time and time again. They don't require any special training and you can start today.

Preventing Heart Disease and Stroke—without Alcohol

DRINKING MODERATE AMOUNTS of alcohol can help to reduce the risk of coronary heart disease and ischemic strokes, but that is not the only approach. In fact, nondrinkers can lower the odds of having a heart attack or stroke without drinking any alcohol at all. Here's how:

• knowledge is power, so ask your physician to monitor your blood cholesterol and blood fat (triglyceride) levels. If your cholesterol or blood fat rises above safe levels, ask your physician what you can do to bring the levels down, and follow that advice carefully
• eat a low-fat diet based on whole grains, fresh vegetables, and fruits
• eat only small amounts of low-fat meat and poultry. Do as Thomas Jefferson did, using meat to flavor your food, rather than as the bulk of your diet
• avoid the saturated fats found in foods such as lard, heavily marbled meats, and deep fried foods
• exercise regularly, at least 30 minutes a day, 3–4 days a week
• maintain your normal weight
• don't smoke
• if you have diabetes, follow your doctor's instructions carefully in order to keep the disease under control
• elevated blood pressure is a risk factor for cardiovascular disease, so ask your physician to monitor your blood pressure. If it's high, ask your doctor what you can do to bring it down, and follow those instructions carefully
• keep your stress to a minimum. Many books have been written on the subject, and you'll find some of them listed in the Bibliography. As you study the literature, you'll find that almost all successful stress-reduction programs can be boiled down to one basic idea: Don't sweat the little things in life, and remember that just about everything is a little thing

GOOD HEALTH IS WITHIN YOUR GRASP

Thanks to mounting scientific evidence pointing to alcohol's advantageous effects on many aspects of health, many physicians and other health experts now agree that alcohol has a role to play in a healthy lifestyle. When taken in moderation and combined with other good health habits, it can help to add years to your life and life to your years. But remember, light-to-moderate consumption of alcohol is but one tool we can use to build good health. The wise builder uses all the available tools, including diet, exercise, stress reduction techniques, and healthy habits.

And those who do not drink need not worry, for they can strengthen their general health and reduce their risk of many diseases without alcohol, simply by following the "Dietary Guidelines For Americans" and incorporating the other good health habits outlined in this chapter.

CHAPTER NINE

Beware of Excess

The benefits of wine are many, if it is taken in the proper amount, as it keeps the body in a healthy condition and cures many illnesses . . . [but] inebriety causes harm."[1]

—MOSES MAIMONIDES, twelfth-century Jewish sage and physician to the Sultan Saladin

MOST PEOPLE HAVE good reasons for enjoying moderate amounts of alcohol: a glass of wine to enhance dinner, a toast to the newlyweds, a beer with a friend at the ball game. For the vast majority of Americans, alcohol is an occasional treat. Unfortunately, a small number of people turn to alcohol for the wrong reasons, drinking when they are angry, embarrassed, worried, upset, or unhappy. They may drink to blot out pain, or perhaps because their friends are doing the same. When that happens, they no longer have good reasons to be drinking.

Overindulgence is an ancient problem. Over two thousand years ago, in the fourth century B.C., members of Alexander the Great's court abused alcohol in drinking contests such as this one described in an ancient manuscript: "Many of the competitors died during the contest or shortly after, but Torquatus Triconglus survived long enough to take the prize, having drunk his twenty-four pints."[2]

Torquatus Triconglus and his fellow alcohol abusers paid the ultimate penalty for drinking to excess. Of course, most abusers don't die immediately. Instead, they suffer through a long series of personal and professional disasters, often harming or destroying family and friends as they spiral downward.

It's An Ancient Problem

ALMOST AS SOON as man discovered the pleasurable effects of alcohol, its side effects were evident. In an ancient Greek work called the *Problemata*,[3] the author wonders:

• why is it that to those who are very drunk everything seems to revolve in a circle?
• why is it that to those who are drunk one thing at which they are looking sometimes appears to be many?
• why is it that those who are drunk are incapable of having sexual intercourse?
• why is it that wine that is mixed but tends toward the unmixed causes a worse headache the next morning than entirely unmixed wine?
• why has wine the effect both of stupefying and of driving to a frenzy those who drink it?
• why is it that cabbage stops the ill effects of drinking?
• why are the drunken more easily moved to tears?
• why is it that the tongues of those who are drunk stumble?
• why is it that oil is beneficial against drunkenness and sipping it enables one to continue drinking?

WHAT IS MODERATE DRINKING?

With drinking, as with most other things in life, moderation is the key. When done in moderation, drinking can make life longer and more enjoyable. In general terms, moderation can be defined as drinking that does not cause physical, mental, emotional, behavioral, social, work-related or other problems. In an attempt to make this vague statement practical, the U.S. Department of Health and Human Services joined with the U.S. Department of Agriculture to offer this definition of moderate drinking in the 1995 "Dietary Guidelines For Americans":

- For most men, no more than two drinks a day
- For most women, no more than one drink a day (One drink consists of 12 ounces of regular beer *or* 5 ounces of wine *or* 1.5 ounces of 80-proof distilled spirits.)

Notice that the guidelines refer to the number of drinks per day, rather than per week or per month. This phrasing is very important. It would have been just as easy to state that men should confine themselves to 14 drinks per week (rather than two per day), but that would suggest that it's reasonable to down all 14 while watching the game on Sunday afternoon, and then have none for the rest of the week. But it's not a good idea to "bank" your alcohol allotment and use it all in one day, for alternating binge drinking and abstention is not healthy. That's why the guidelines specifically state no more than two drinks *per day* for men, and one *per day* for women.

These are, of course, just guidelines. Some people can drink more without having any problems, while others must limit themselves to less—or none at all. If you're not sure whether you can drink a little more or less than the guidelines suggest, err on the side of caution and opt for less.

And then there are those who, according to the government guidelines, should not drink at all, under any circumstances, at any time:

- children and adolescents
- those who have trouble limiting themselves to moderate consumption
- pregnant women, or women who are trying to conceive
- anyone planning to engage in activities, such as driving, that require skill or attention within the next several hours or more
- anyone under the age of twenty-one
- alcoholics or recovering alcoholics

And of course, anyone taking medicines of any kind should check with a physician to make sure that the medication will not adversely interact with alcohol.

There are other people who should think carefully before drinking. It's possible that alcohol could exaggerate the effects of manic depression or other mental illnesses in some people, so people with psychiatric disorders may be wise to abstain. Those with compulsive disorders may also need to say "no thanks" to drinking, rather than risk overdoing it.

A DRINKING PROBLEM?

How much drinking is too much? When does a pleasant activity become an addiction? The National Council on Alcoholism and Drug Dependence has defined alcoholism as *"a primary, chronic disease with genetic, psychosocial and environmental factors influencing its development and manifestation. The disease is often progressive and fatal. It is characterized by impaired control over drinking, preoccupation with the drug alcohol, use of alcohol despite adverse consequences, and distortions in thinking, most notably denial. Each of these symptoms may be continuous or periodic."* In other words, the alcoholic is preoccupied with drinking, and continues drinking despite adverse consequences to his or her physical, mental, or emotional health or to his or her family, professional, or social life. Other authorities simply say that if you can drink enough to raise your blood alcohol level to .300 or greater, you have a problem.

The American Psychiatric Association divides problem drinkers into three categories, according to the abuse patterns they adopt: heavy drinking every day, heavy drinking on weekends or other times when they have no work responsibilities, or long periods of sobriety interrupted by "binges" or "benders."[4] Whatever the pattern or the cause, problem drinkers should be quickly identified and helped. Here are some of the signs that one has, or may be developing, a drinking problem:

- *getting drunk*—Although becoming inebriated is not in itself a sign of alcoholism, it does indicate that you've gone past your limit. The more frequently you drink to drunkenness, the greater the danger of developing a drinking problem
- *drinking in anticipation of stressful situations or drinking to forget*—When alcohol becomes a crutch, rather than an accompaniment to life's pleasures, it is being abused
- *drinking and driving*—One who chooses to ignore the well-known dangers of drinking and driving has lost the ability to reason and plan ahead
- *drinking before working, going to school, or performing other important daily tasks*—Alcohol has either become a way to help one

through difficult situations, or is so important that one is willing to risk failure in order to keep drinking

- *drinking in the morning*—Needing an "eye opener" suggests that you can't get through the day without help from the bottle
- *letting drinking interfere with work, relationships, and other aspects of life*—Problem drinkers may make everything else in their lives secondary to their next drink
- *being unable to enjoy yourself socially unless you've had a few "belts"*—Feeling comfortable with others only when you're "buzzed" or drunk indicates a serious problem
- *Becoming angry, loud or, violent when drinking*—If this happens, then drinking is enhancing the darker side of your personality and allowing it to "come out"
- *drinking alone*—Moderate drinkers tend to share a drink with friends, or use alcohol to celebrate important events or days. Drinking alone is, by definition, not a social event
- *spending time with other heavy drinkers*—Drinking with other heavy drinkers loosens the restraints one might impose on oneself when with moderate or nondrinkers
- *planning when and where to get the next drink*—Those who plan their schedules around that next drink are obsessed with alcohol
- *denying drinking, or lying about how much you've consumed*—You hope to avoid being pressured to take care of your problem, and you deny your problem to yourself and others
- *changing your behavior in order to drink*—Problem drinkers may lie, cheat, or do whatever else is necessary to continue drinking. Drinking is all that matters to them.
- *hiding alcohol at home and/or work, or sneaking away to grab a "quick one"*—Fear of letting others know how much you are drinking and when, indicates that you know your drinking is inappropriate, but are unable to control yourself
- *"needing" a drink at any time during the day or night*—Enjoying a cocktail or a glass of wine with dinner, or a beer during the game, is quite different than feeling compelled to have another drink, right now! When you reach this stage, you are probably addicted
- *forgetting how much alcohol you've consumed*
- *suffering from frequent hangovers*
- *suffering from "blackouts"*—When you have no idea what you were doing while you were drunk, it's definitely time to seek help
- *suffering from the "D.T.'s"*—Delirium tremens is a sign of severe

107

physical distress due to excessive and prolonged use of alcohol, characterized by restlessness, agitation, disorientation, mental confusion, hallucinations, fear, trembling of the hands and other physical, mental, and emotional symptoms. (See box on page 109)

As with other diseases, alcoholism is easier to treat in the early stages before it consumes you physically, mentally, and emotionally. If you have any of these symptoms, or have any reason to suspect that you have a drinking problem, get help immediately.

ALCOHOL, GENETICS, AND UPBRINGING

There's a great deal of controversy over the causes of alcoholism. Some researchers feel that alcoholism is a learned behavior. Others contend that alcoholism, or at least the tendency toward alcoholism, is passed down from generation to generation via the genes. To bolster their argument, they'll point to studies that have found that when adopted children grow up, their drinking habits are much more like those of one of the biologic parents than either of their adoptive parents.

The "nature versus nurture" debate will continue for some time. It is, however, safe to say that genetics as well as cultural, family, and psychological factors help to determine whether or not we will become problem drinkers. But since we have absolutely no control over our genetic inheritances, and precious little over our childhood environments, we should monitor ourselves and our behavior carefully, watching for the signs of danger. These signs include:

- a family history of alcoholism
- reacting "differently" to alcohol—If it takes much less alcohol to make you "happy" or to put you to sleep than it does others, you may be more susceptible to the drink than others. On the other hand, it's also a bad sign if you can drink prodigious quantities of alcohol without suffering any ill effects—and the sheer volume consumed may be damaging your body
- setting limits for yourself, then often going beyond
- deciding to stop drinking, but being unable to do so
- switching from one drink to another, looking for the one that won't make you drunk

The D.T.'s—a Sure Sign of Excess

DELIRIUM TREMENS, CALLED the "D.T.'s" for short, is a serious, possibly fatal reaction to the prolonged, excessive consumption of alcohol. The D.T.'s may strike after a long binge of heavy drinking and poor eating, or may come during a period of abstinence. They may be triggered by an infection or injury to the head or appear as "withdrawal" symptoms after a long period of drinking.

Symptoms of the D.T.'s include restlessness, agitation, disorientation, mental confusion, hallucinations, fear, poor appetite, difficulty sleeping, excitement agitation, anxiety, heavy perspiration, stomach upset, chest pain, a very rapid heartbeat, and tremors of the hands, feet, legs, and tongue. A "D.T. attack" can last up to six days. If the problem is not treated, symptoms can progress to respiratory infections, pneumonia, extreme fatigue, severe dehydration, and heart failure. Those suffering from delirium tremens may also have serious nutritional deficiencies, which can trigger a host of other problems. If and when the doctors are able to solve the physical symptoms of the D.T.'s, the alcoholic will still have to deal with the remorse and depression that often follows. Unfortunately, suicides are not uncommon.

- envying those who can "hold their liquor" better than you can
- wishing that others would stop telling you that you drink too much
- needing to start the day off with a drink
- having trouble at home, work, or school, or in personal or social relationships because of drinking
- wishing that you could stop drinking
- suffering from blackouts

Numerous doctors, psychologists, and medical facilities all across the country stand ready to help problem drinkers. They have a wide array of treatments, including such traditional psychological and medical approaches as behavior therapy, aversion therapy, and the use of Antabuse, and other medicines. One of the best-known and perhaps the most successful treatment organizations is Alcoholics Anonymous, a loosely knit "fellowship" of men and women who share their experiences and help each other.

Alcoholics Anonymous began informally in Akron, Ohio, back in 1935, with the meeting of two alcoholics, one a stockbroker and the other a physician. Both men had been associated with a spiritually based nonalcoholic society called the Oxford Group. Together, they helped put a patient at Akron City Hospital on the road to recovery from alcoholism. These three men then formed what was later known as Alcoholics Anonymous. With a program based on the now well-known "Twelve Steps," Alcoholics Anonymous has thousands of chapters around the world. It costs nothing to join. Membership is open to anyone who sincerely wishes to break free of problem drinking or addiction. New members are sponsored or guided by experienced members, and can call upon others for help when necessary. The heart of Alcoholics Anonymous lies in the Twelve Steps, which recap what the group's earliest members learned about themselves. The Twelve Steps urge members to:

- admit that they have no power to handle alcohol or its effects, and that alcohol has made their lives unmanageable
- understand that only a Higher Power can restore normalcy to their lives
- ask God, however God is understood, to take control of their lives
- carefully, relentlessly examine their moral underpinnings, including their shortcomings and failures
- tell themselves, others, and God what they have done wrong
- prepare themselves to ask God to correct their character and moral flaws
- ask God to correct these flaws
- think about the people they have harmed, and be willing to do whatever it takes to right those wrongs
- go ahead and right those wrongs, unless doing so would hurt someone

- keep examining their moral underpinnings, identifying and admitting to any errors
- communicate with God through prayer and other means, asking God what he wants them to do, and to give them the power to follow through
- help teach other alcoholics how to help themselves

Alcoholics Anonymous emphasizes that the disease of alcoholism does not usually disappear or regress on its own. Instead, it gets progressively worse and can never be cured, for an alcoholic is always an alcoholic and is always in danger of "falling off in the wagon." But alcoholics *can* learn to control the problem by completely abstaining from alcohol and by practicing the Twelve Steps.

Alcoholics Anonymous groups are located all over the country. Local chapters are listed in the phone book. You can find a list of chapters, via the Internet, on the Alcoholics Anonymous home page at: http://www.alcoholics-anonymous.org/index.html

What You Think When You Drink Makes a Difference

DOES DRINKING AFFECT all people the same way? Individual reactions are impossible to predict, but a look at the way large groups of people respond to alcohol suggests that what we're taught about drinking (and getting drunk) plays a major role in modifying our behavior.

According to David Pittman, Professor Emeritus of Psychology at St. Louis's Washington University,[5] cultures adopt one of four attitudes toward drinking:

- *abstinence*—an abhorrence of alcohol, often for religious reasons. The Islamic and Hindu cultures embrace abstinence

continued

• *permissiveness*—an acceptance of moderate consumption at prescribed times, such as during meals. Drinking is considered an important adjunct to meals and festivals, a social lubricant and/or a sign of hospitality. Children are often allowed to partake of small or moderate amounts of alcohol during meals or religious services. But while moderate drinking is condoned, antisocial behavior while under the influence of alcohol is not. Permissiveness is found in Greece, Italy, Spain, France, and other countries. American Jews also have a permissive attitude toward drinking. They begin to drink at an early age as part of religious and social ceremonies, but do not tolerate drunkenness

• *ambivalence*—a love/hate relationship with alcohol. Alcohol is considered bad, but drinking inevitable. Alcohol is kept from the young until a certain age, then it is suddenly not only permissible but "cool." Adults who can "hold their liquor" are admired. Bad behavior while under the influence is simultaneously condemned and condoned. Over-imbibers are expected to become belligerent or violent, and women who drink are thought to be signaling sexual receptiveness. Many gatherings are held for the sole purpose of drinking or drinking to excess. The United States has a ambivalent attitude toward alcohol. Professor Pittman feels that this ambivalent attitude toward alcohol, focusing on the extremes (abstinence and drunkenness), prevents us from developing more moderate and stable attitudes toward drinking. He notes that our attitude "restricts the meaning of drinking to one of hedonism . . . drinking becomes an extreme and uncontrolled behavior for many."[6]

• *overpermissiveness*—both overconsumption and antisocial behavior while drunk are expected and tolerated.

It appears that what we're taught about alcohol plays a large role in determining how much we consume, and what we do while drinking. If we've been taught that the "demon rum" will destroy our morals and make us violent, we're more likely to exhibit bad behavior when drinking. If, on the other hand, we've learned that alcohol makes people more friendly and gregarious, and that drunken riotousness is bad, we're more likely to behave ourselves when imbibing.

The Careful Drinker

To ensure that you are a careful, responsible drinker, remember the following:

- only drink because *you* want to, not because it's "time" to drink, others are drinking, or a drink has been placed in your hand
- plan ahead so that you won't have to drive home after drinking
- know your limit, and decide beforehand when you will stop
- keep track of everything you drink. Don't accept a glass unless you know how much alcohol it contains
- eat before you begin drinking. The fat and protein in foods can help to slow the passage of alcohol from your stomach and intestines to your bloodstream
- pace yourself. Drink small amounts of alcohol at a time, rather than a lot at once. Sip, rather than gulp. Remember, the point is to enjoy the beverage, not to get drunk. And never participate in "chugging" contests or vie with others to see who can consume the most in the least amount of time
- develop strategies to deal with others who "push" you to drink more. The best approach is to simply say "No, thank you, I've had enough." If you're uncomfortable doing that, hold a glass of orange juice, cola, water, or another nonalcoholic beverage. This will make them think that you're drinking
- stop drinking or switch to nonalcoholic beverages before the gathering breaks up. This will give your liver time to burn up some of the alcohol you've consumed
- stop when you reach your predetermined limit. It doesn't matter what time it is or how much more partying remains ahead. When you hit your limit, stop
- never urge others to drink if they don't want to
- never drink alcoholic beverages to quench your thirst. If you're thirsty, you need water.
- be sure to discuss your drinking habits with your physician or pharmacist before taking any prescription or nonprescription medicines. Unless you get a specific "Okay" to continue drinking while taking the medicines, abstain

If you're hosting a gathering at which alcoholic beverages are served, be sure to offer food right away, before the drinking starts. Have plenty of soda, juice, sparkling water, and other nonalcoholic beverages. Never press a drink on anyone, and don't run around topping off every drink you see. As the host, you set the tone. You play a large role in helping your guests to drink moderately.

With Medicine Like This, Who Needs a Drink?

SOME MEDICATIONS CONTAIN a surprising amount of alcohol, which may explain why they are so popular. Here's a quick list of the alcohol content of some common remedies:

Medicine	Percent Alcohol
Nyquil	25.0
Cepacol Mouthwash	14.0
Dristan Cold Formula	12.0
Geritol Liquid	12.0
Contact JR	10.0
Tylenol Cold	7.5
Chlor-Trimeton Syrup	7.0
Tylenol Drops	7.0
Senokot Syrup	7.0
Fergon	6.0
Dramamine Junior Syrup	5.0
Triaminic	5.0
Robitussin CF	4.8
Robitussin (plain)	3.5
Sudafed Liquid	3.0
Dimetane Elixir	3.0
Dimetapp Elixir	2.3
Robitussin DM	1.4
Robitussin PE	1.4

CHAPTER TEN

Alcohol Q&A

What is alcohol?

WHEN WE SPEAK of alcohol we usually mean ethyl alcohol, also known as ethanol, the primary alcohol found in alcoholic beverages. It's a clear and colorless liquid with a relatively simple chemical structure. Ethyl alcohol has various effects on the mind and body.

What are some other types of alcohol?

There's also methyl alcohol (used in cleansers and solvents), isopropyl alcohol (the kind doctors use), and denatured alcohol. Denatured alcohol, which is used in antifreeze and other products, is ethyl alcohol that has been mixed with other substances to make it taste and smell bad. It's deliberately contaminated so people won't drink it.

What effects does alcohol have on the body?

Alcohol is a local anesthetic, an irritant, and a sedative. Even in small amounts, it can induce lightheadedness and dizziness, it depresses the central nervous system, lowers inhibitions, alters behavior, changes the mood, makes the heart beat faster, increases sweating, changes the body's temperature, irritates the stomach lining, and increases urination. By lowering inhibitions it may increase sexual desires, but it can also cause temporary impotence.

How rapidly is the alcohol you drink absorbed into the bloodstream?

That depends on many factors, including how much is consumed in a given amount of time, the size of your body, your metabolism, and the amount and type of food and fluid already in your stomach. Your sex is also important, for alcohol tends to affect women faster, more intensely, and longer than it does men. The concentration of alcohol in the blood peaks between 60 and 90 minutes after drinking, then begins to taper off as it is converted by the liver into carbon dioxide and water.

Is there any way to slow the absorption?

Eat before drinking, especially fatty foods, and drink slowly.

How quickly can the liver "burn off" alcohol?

It varies from person to person, but averages about 8 to 9 grams per hour—less than the amount found in one standard drink.

What is the blood alcohol level?

Often called BAC, the blood alcohol level measures how many grams of alcohol there are in every 100 milliliters of a person's blood. A BAC of 0.02–0.08 can cause mood changes, altered behavior, and impaired coordination. A BAC of 0.100–0.199 can cause poor judgment, slowed reaction time, plus trouble standing and walking steadily. A BAC of 0.200–0.299 can cause vomiting. A BAC of 0.300 can cause blackouts. A BAC of 0.400 or more can cause alcohol poisoning, coma, and death.

Does everyone behave the same way when drinking?

No. Alcohol has predictable effects on human physiology, but our attitudes toward drinking and drunkenness influence our behaviors when we are drinking. Our expectations and past experiences with alcohol play a role, as do why, with whom, where, and when we are drinking. One who expects to behave properly when drinking will probably do much better than one who drinks the same amount but *expects* to become drunk and obnoxious.

Is there any way to cure a hangover?

Sauerkraut juice, B vitamins, and pure oxygen have all been tried, but the best cure is not to drink, or certainly not to drink past your limit.

Is alcohol nutritious?

Not particularly. Alcoholic beverages have small and variable amounts of B vitamins, potassium, calcium, magnesium, and other vitamins and minerals. Wine also contains resveratrol and other healthful phytochemicals. Beer is perhaps the most nutritious of the alcoholic beverages, but even a full quart does not provide a significant portion of the Recommended Dietary Allowance for any vitamin or mineral.

Does drinking always lead to a "beer belly?"

No. Alcohol does have calories (7 calories per gram, compared to 9 calories per gram for fat, and 4 calories per gram for protein and carbohydrate), and these calories, like calories from any other foods or drinks, can make us heavier if consumed in excess. But there's nothing extra fattening about alcohol. In fact, some researchers have suggested that regularly drinking small amounts of alcohol may help people control their weight.

What is a "standard" drink?

A standard drink contains 10–12 grams (½ ounce) of ethyl alcohol, the amount found in 12 ounces of regular beer *or* 5 ounces of wine *or* 1.5 ounces of 80-proof distilled spirits. These drinks are equivalent in the sense that they all contain the same amount of alcohol.

How much alcohol is in a typical drink?

It varies from brand to brand, but in general, beer is about 4.5–5.5 percent alcohol, with some "light" beers having less and malt beverages more. Most table wines are 10–12 percent alcohol, with fortified wine containing 14 percent or more. Many spirits are 35 or 37 percent alcohol, with stronger brands containing 40 percent. A few spirits run as high as 50 percent alcohol and even higher.

What is the difference between percent alcohol and proof?

A drink's "proof" is almost exactly double its alcohol content. A beer containing 5 percent alcohol is 10 proof.

Alcohol has been featured on 60 Minutes, Time Magazine, *and just about everywhere else in the past five or so years. Why all the hoopla?*

Researchers became interested in the "French Paradox" in the early 1990s. It seems that the French eat much more fat than we do and they don't exercise nearly as much as we do, yet they have far less coronary heart disease. That's the paradox: Why do they have healthier hearts, despite their unhealthy behaviors? Many feel that the answer lies in all the wine the French drink. Something in wine or other alcoholic beverages must protect them against coronary heart disease.

How does alcohol protect against coronary heart disease?

A great many studies have shown that light-to-moderate consumption of alcohol can protect the heart in several ways, including increasing the beneficial HDL cholesterol, "thinning" the blood, lowering blood pressure, and reducing stress.

What is HDL?

HDL stands for high-density lipoprotein, a "type" of cholesterol. It's called the "good" cholesterol because it helps to keep the arteries clear. Higher HDL levels, 45 or more, are considered protective. A low HDL level is considered a risk factor for heart disease.

Is it possible to increase the HDL?

Exercise has long been considered the best method of pushing up the HDL. Many studies have also found that drinking small to moderate amounts of alcohol can increase the HDL. It apparently only takes a few weeks before careful drinking pushes up the HDL.

Is the alcohol-induced rise in HDL significant?

Yes. Results of the "MR. FIT," Honolulu Heart, and LRC Follow-Up studies suggest that about half of alcohol's protective effects on the heart can be attributed to the alcohol-induced increase in HDL.

Why is alcohol's ability to "thin" the blood beneficial?

The blood clots that can become lodged in narrowed arteries in the heart or brain, triggering a heart attack or ischemic stroke, are less likely to form if the blood is "thin." (You don't want the blood to be too thin, of course. Otherwise it could not properly clot when you cut yourself.) Studies have found that drinking moderate amounts of alcohol for just a few weeks can make the blood "thinner" and less "sticky," thus reducing the risk of heart disease and stroke caused by clots.

How is blood pressure related to heart disease and alcohol?

Elevated blood pressure (hypertension) is considered a major risk factor for coronary heart disease. The results of several studies suggest that light to moderate amounts of alcohol lower blood pressure, which in turn reduces the risk of suffering a heart attack. Beware, however for heavy drinking can *raise* blood pressure

How does reducing stress protect against heart disease?

The new medical science called psychoneuroimmunology has shown that stress can elevate cholesterol, cause coronary arteries to "clamp down," and fill the body with powerful chemicals that jolt the heart (as well as the immune system and the rest of the body). Light-to-moderate consumption helps to reduce anxiety and tension, making it a useful weapon in the fight against stress. It also helps to relieve depression, tension, and self-consciousness, helping many people to become more sociable. This is very important, for pleasantly interacting with others is a great way to relieve stress.

To what extent does alcohol aid the heart? A little or a lot?

The results of many studies conducted in research centers across the United States and Europe and reported in prestigious medical journals, suggest that moderate consumption of wine, beer, or spirits can reduce the risk of dying from fatal heart attacks by 10–70 percent. But remember, these are only statistics drawn from large groups of people. No one can say exactly how much you will benefit, if at all.

How much does one have to drink to help the heart?

One to two drinks per day is enough. In fact, the United States government defines moderate drinking as 2 standard drinks per day for men, and 1 a day for women.

If some alcohol is good, is more better?

Absolutely not! Heavy drinking will damage your heart, as well as the rest of your body and your mind. Moderation is the key to drinking, as it is with most things in life.

Is drinking the only way to help the heart?

No, you needn't drink a drop. A healthful diet, regular exercise, stress reduction, and good lifestyle habits can help you reduce your risk of coronary artery disease—quite significantly.

Still, is it a good idea to drink to protect the heart?

Light-to-moderate consumption of alcohol has beneficial effects on the heart, but that's not a good reason to begin drinking, or to increase consumption. If you're interested in a healthy heart, look to diet, exercise, stress reduction, and good lifestyle habits.

Is there any difference, as far as heart health is concerned, between beer, wine, and liquor?

No. Despite the presence of resveratrol and other phytochemicals in wine, the best evidence to date suggests that it's the ethanol in all types of alcoholic beverages that can improve one's health. Perhaps future studies will pinpoint specific health benefits of the different beverages.

What is the relationship between alcohol and stroke?

Light-to-moderate consumption of alcohol reduces the risk of blockage strokes in much the same way that it works against coronary heart disease. It increases the levels of the "good" HDL cholesterol, "thins" the blood to prevent the formation of unnecessary blood clots that can lodge in an artery in the brain, and reduces the odds of a sudden spasm of the smooth muscle that wraps around the cerebral arteries.

*Is it a good idea to drink a lot of alcohol as a "medicine"
against strokes?*

No. Several researchers have found that light drinking can protect
against ischemic ("blockage") strokes, but more than a couple of
drinks a day increases the odds of suffering from a hemorrhagic ("rupture") stroke. Binge drinking also increases the risk of stroke.

How does alcohol help stress?

Physicians have long known that a little bit of alcohol helps many of
those suffering from stress or depression. Light-to-moderate drinking
can reduce stress, increase happiness, affective expression, and conviviality, reduce tension, depression, and self-consciousness, boost certain types of cognitive (thinking) performance, and help with some of
the psychiatric problems associated with aging and illness.

In that case should we drink when we're stressed?

No. You should never use alcoholic beverages as a medicine. There
are many excellent stress-reduction techniques that can be used instead.

Does alcohol raise blood pressure?

Along with obesity, heredity, gender, race, and diet, the consumption
of more than 30 to 60 grams of alcohol a day is considered a major
risk factor for hypertension. Light-to-moderate consumption, however, is not believed to be a risk factor. In fact, light consumption may
actually *lower* blood pressure in some people.

Should diabetics avoid alcohol?

Several studies have shown that alcohol can help diabetics keep their
blood sugar levels under control. And light-to-moderate consumption
also raises the HDL ("good") cholesterol. This is especially important
for diabetics, who are at increased risk of heart disease. However, all
diabetics should consult their doctors before drinking alcoholic beverages.

Does alcohol aid digestion?

Many people consider alcohol to be a digestive aid. It stimulates salivation, and protects against certain food-borne bacteria. Be careful, however, for heavy drinking can damage the lining of the stomach.

Does alcohol prevent gallstones?

Studies have shown that moderate drinking may prevent cholesterol gallstones by lowering the bile cholesterol saturation. *Excessive* drinking, however, is believed to increase the risk.

Does alcohol cause cancer?

Although ethyl alcohol is not a carcinogen, it appears to act as a co-carcinogen, "strengthening" other cancer-causing factors. Drinking can increase the risk of developing cancers of the mouth, esophagus, and other parts of the body, including possibly the breast, colon, and rectum. If you have a family history of cancer, if you smoke, if you consume a high-fat diet, or have any other risk factors for cancer, it is best to abstain.

Is it safe for senior citizens to drink?

As long as they have no health problems that may be worsened by drinking, and if they are not taking medicines that interact adversely with alcohol, there is no reason that most seniors cannot enjoy moderate imbibing. In fact, small amounts of alcohol can help improve the appetite and bowel function, lift the mood, increase sociability, and relieve stress in certain oldsters. But alcohol can worsen memory problems and interfere with sleep, so drinking should be done with caution and in moderation only.

Does alcohol improve our overall health?

Light-to-moderate drinkers tend to be hospitalized less often than either abstainers or heavy drinkers. This suggests that alcohol contributes to overall well-being (or at least to the feeling that one is healthier).

Does drinking extend our lives?

The Framingham Study, the Japanese Physician's Study, the British Regional Heart Study, the American Cancer Study, the Kaiser Permanente Study, the Brusselton Study, the British Doctor's Study and others have shown that light-to-moderate drinking can reduce the odds of death from all causes. The positive results of these studies have been consistent with different ethnic and age groups and both sexes.

Let me be clear about one thing: The risk of death due to auto accidents and some other causes *rises* with alcohol consumption. It's only because the death rate due to coronary heart disease and other problems drops so dramatically that the *overall risk of death* falls among light and moderate imbibers.

Should one drink?

The evidence is strong and clear: light-to-moderate consumption of alcohol can reduce the risk of coronary heart disease, and ischemic stroke, relieve stress, improve other aspects of health, and reduce the overall risk of death. But alcohol is not a magic cure, and it does have disadvantages. Even small amounts pose risks for some people, and the dangers of heavy drinking are well known.

Overall, it's safe to say that careful drinking as part of a healthy lifestyle can promote health in many people. However, one should not begin drinking or drink more just to get these health benefits. You can do the same by improving your diet, exercising more, reducing your stress, and adopting healthy lifestyle habits.

What is the government's position on alcohol?

In January 1996, the United States government stated, for the first time ever, that light-to-moderate drinking could be a health aid, and that alcohol had a role to play in a healthy diet and lifestyle.

If I wanted to reduce my risk of heart disease and stroke without drinking alcohol, how would I go about it?

There are many things you can do, including the following: Keep your cholesterol and blood fats (triglycerides) within safe limits, eat a low-fat diet, eat plenty of fresh vegetables and fruits and whole grains, avoid saturated fats, exercise regularly, maintain normal weight, refrain from smoking, monitor your blood pressure and keep it under control should it rise, carefully follow your doctor's instructions should you have diabetes, and keep your stress to a minimum.

What, besides alcohol, reduces stress?

There are many ways to relieve stress, including taking life a little slower, relaxing every day, having fun every day, exercising regularly, meditating, taking part in family activities, joining social and neighborhood organizations, helping others, only planning to do as much as you comfortably can every day, acting and walking and talking enthusiastically, looking upon problems as exciting challenges, and believing in yourself.

One final question. How good is the alcohol-health evidence?

Most new ideas are controversial, for they challenge the "old order." Fortunately, the alcohol-health studies have been published in some of the most respected and prestigious medical and scientific journals in the world, including the *Journal of the American Medical Association, Lancet, Annals of Internal Medicine,* the *American Journal of Cardiology,* the *British Medical Journal,* the *International Journal of Epidemiology,* and the *American Journal of Epidemiology.* The fact that the studies have appeared in journals of this caliber suggests that the evidence is indeed strong.

Appendix 1
Alcohol and the Heart in the Medical Literature

THE IDEA THAT alcohol can be good for you is startling. Like all ideas that challenge what we "know," this one faces opposition. The best way to overcome well-intentioned skepticism is to lay out the evidence. We can't possibly review all the alcohol/health studies in this book, so I've decided to focus on the alcohol/heart connection, gathering together many of the studies in this appendix. These are not the only alcohol/heart studies, and are not necessarily the "best." I've chosen these studies because they demonstrate the depth and breadth of the information available and because, frankly, they intrigue me.

REPETITION STRENGTHENS SCIENTIFIC ARGUMENTS

You'll see a lot of what appears to be repetition in these studies. That's because many of the studies are designed to investigate the same issue from slightly different angles. The more that researchers who are working independently in separate laboratories around the world, each with their own biases and agendas and ideas, are able to come to the same conclusion, the stronger the overall argument. And so you'll read about researchers using different groups of subjects, different methods, differing lengths of time, different amounts of alcohol, et cetera. Each study that comes to the same conclusion using different methods strengthens the proof.

Remember ...

A STANDARD DRINK contains 10 grams (½ ounce) of alcohol, the amount found in a 5-ounce glass of wine, a 12-ounce can of beer, or a single serving of spirits (1¼–1½ ounces).

DOES ALCOHOL PROTECT THE HEART?

The key question, the one that must be answered first, is whether there is any scientific proof that alcohol (specifically the ethyl alcohol, or ethanol, found in alcoholic beverages) protects the heart. Here's the summary of an important early research project that said "yes."

STUDY SUMMARY: Earlier analysis of the information collected in Kaiser Permanente studies found that regular alcohol consumption reduced the risk of heart attacks. A new study of hospitalizations confirmed that those drinking up to two alcoholic beverages per day have less cardiovascular disease than either abstainers or heavy drinkers.

CITATION: Klatsky, A. L., Friedman G. D., Siegelaub A. B., "Alcohol Use and Cardiovascular Disease: The Kaiser Permanente Experience" *Circulation* 64 (suppl. III): 32–41 (1981)

Other early evidence came from overseas. Here's the synopsis of a study involving 10,000 Yugoslavian men. The men were enlisted to help researchers examine the relationship between drinking and non-sudden death from coronary heart disease.

STUDY SUMMARY: Consumption of alcoholic beverages was inversely related to non-sudden coronary death. This means that as alcohol consumption increased (to a certain point), the risk of dying of heart disease dropped. The greatest protective benefit was found in the moderate drinkers.

CITATION: Kozarevic, D., et al., "Drinking Habits and Death: The Yugoslavian Cardiovascular Disease Study" *International Journal of Epidemiology* 12 (2): 145–150 (1983).

Back in the United States, civil servants in New York State provided more early confirmation of the beneficial link between alcohol and heart disease.

STUDY SUMMARY: Examinations were conducted and drinking histories were obtained from 1,755 men in 1953–54. The men ranged in age from 38–55, and almost all (1708) were free of heart disease. The men were examined at various times through the years, and another alcohol consumption history was obtained in 1971–72. There were two follow-up periods; the first covering 18 years, the second 10 years. RESULTS: The results at the end of the first follow-up period were not statically significant. At the end of the second follow-up period, however, it was clear that consuming alcohol lowered the risk of coronary heart disease.

CITATION: Doyle, J. T., Gordon, T., Drinking and Coronary Heart Disease: The Albany Study, *American Heart Journal* 110 (2): 331–334 (1985).

Perhaps the most famous and prestigious long-term study of health in America is the Framingham Heart Study. The effects of alcohol on coronary heart disease were examined in the original Framingham study, beginning in 1948. Data from the study support the argument that light-to-moderate consumption of alcohol can be cardioprotective. The alcohol/heart information derived from Framingham was published in the *American Journal of Epidemiology* in 1986.

RESULTS FOR MEN: In both the raw data and the Cox regression analyses, alcohol produced a U-shaped relationship with respect to death from coronary heart disease in male nonsmokers and heavy smokers. That is, beginning with abstainers at the top left of the U, the risk of death from coronary artery disease for light and moderate drinkers fell. (You can trace the drop by moving your eye down along the left side of the U.) As alcohol consumption moved into the heavy range, however, the risk began rising again (to complete the U). Consumption of alcoholic beverages was subdivided into beer, wine, and spirits, with all three showing a strong U curve for nonsmokers and heavy smokers. In nonsmokers, however, beer and wine appeared to do a better job of protecting against deaths from coronary heart disease than did spirits.

RESULTS FOR WOMEN: Alcohol consumption did not lower the risk of dying of heart disease among nonsmokers. The data suggested a U-shaped curve of protective effect for smokers, but the Cox analysis could not confirm this.

CITATION: Kimball, A. W., Friedman, L. A., "Coronary Heart Disease Mortality and Alcohol Consumption in Framingham" *American Journal of Epidemiology* 124 (3): 481–489 (1986).

The same year saw the publication of another study backing the idea that moderate consumption of alcohol protects the heart. In this 1986 study, also published in the *American Journal of Epidemiology,* residents of Washington state served as test subjects.

STUDY SUMMARY: Researchers examined 152 people who had suffered from primary cardiac arrest (heart attack) during the 14 months between December 1979 and January 1981 in Washington's King County. The subjects ranged in age from 25–75, and had not had prior heart disease. 152 other residents of King County, with similar demographics, were used as a control group. Spouses were interviewed to find out how much alcohol the subjects and controls had consumed during the previous year. RESULTS: Drinking light-to-moderate amounts of alcohol produced a reduced risk of suffering primary cardiac arrest. This was true even after accounting for the effects of elevated blood pressure, smoking, and physical activity. Compared to nondrinkers and those who consumed less than one drink per month, moderate drinkers (1–3 drinks per day) had only about half the risk of suffering a heart attack.

CITATION: Siscovick, D. S., "Moderate Alcohol Consumption and Primary Cardiac Arrest" *American Journal of Epidemiology* 123: 499–503 (1986).

Medical researchers from Australia added this study to the medical literature in 1987. Like the Yugoslavian study, it showed that the cardioprotective effects of alcohol were not confined to the United States, and were not a statistical quirk caused by some uniquely American dietary, lifestyle, or other habits.

STUDY SUMMARY: This study was performed to determine the effects of regular exercise and alcoholic beverages on fatal and nonfatal heart attacks in men and women in Auckland, New Zealand. RESULTS: Compared to nondrinkers, those who drank alcohol were less likely to suffer from fatal or nonfatal heart attacks. Physical activity also lowered the risk, but only in those who had been exercising for at least five years.

CITATION: Scragg, R., et al., "Alcohol and Exercise in Myocardial Infarction and Sudden Coronary Death in Men and Women" *American Journal of Epidemiology* 126 (1): 77–85 (1987).

The Trinidad Survey followed 1,341 men for many years. The results of this study, which were published in the *International Journal of Epidemiology,* support the argument that moderate consumption of alcohol is cardioprotective.

STUDY SUMMARY: The 1,341 Trinidadian men, ranging in age from 35–69, were studied in the 1970s and 1980s. During the course of the study, heart disease, artery disease, and/or diabetes increased in 118 of the men, who had previously been heavy drinkers. They were excluded, along with anyone else who had coronary heart disease or diabetes when the study began. RESULTS: The amount of alcohol consumed during the week before they entered the study was inversely related to the mens' risk of coronary heart disease during the course of follow-up (which averaged 7.5 years). Even after age, ethnicity, smoking habits, blood pressure, and serum cholesterol were accounted for, the ones who consumed 5.14 drinks had roughly half the risk of the abstainers.

Miller, G. J., et al., "Alcohol Consumption: Protection against Coronary Heart Disease and Risks to Health" *International Journal of Epidemiology* 19 (4): 923–30 (1990).

Even more positive information was derived from a major study, one often quoted in the scientific and popular literature: The National Health And Nutrition Examination Survey, also known as NHANES I, and the NHANES I Follow-Up. This 1993 study, published in the *American Journal of Public Health,* utilized information from NHANES I and the NHANES I Follow-Up to see if drinking alcohol had a positive effect on heart health.

STUDY SUMMARY: Data derived from the NHANES I, which was conducted between 1971 and 1974, and NHANES I Follow-Up, which ran between 1982 and 1984, was sifted through in an effort to determine if moderate drinking reduced coronary heart disease deaths among White men and women. The authors found that moderate alcohol consumption had a beneficial effect on White men. They noted that statistical models showed 3–4 percent increase in life span for moderate drinkers, compared to light drinkers or abstainers.

CITATION: Coate, D., "Moderate Drinking and Coronary Heart Disease Mortality: Evidence from NHANES I and the NHANES I Follow-Up" *American Journal of Public Health* 83 (6): 888–90 (June 1993).

Intrigued by the "French Paradox," two researchers from the University of California studied information on diet, alcohol, and deaths from 21 developed, relatively affluent countries. This multination study again confirmed that alcohol's cardioprotective effects were not limited to the United States, or any other country. Their findings were reported in the prestigious British journal *Lancet* in 1994.

STUDY SUMMARY: Data from 1954, 1970, 1980, and 1988 was examined, with the consumption of wine, beer, and liquor assessed individually to see which type of alcohol, if any, had the most beneficial effects. The strongest and most consistent relationship the researchers found was the inverse relationship between ethanol from wine and coronary heart disease. In other words, an increased consumption of wine (up to a certain point) produced a decreased risk of heart disease. They did not find, however, that wine increased longevity.

CITATION: Criqui, M. H., Ringel, B. L., "Does Diet or Alcohol Explain the French Paradox?" *Lancet* 344 (8939–8940): 1719–23 (24–31 December 1994).

Scotland chimed in with a major study of its own in 1995, published in the *Journal of Epidemiology and Community Health*. The Scottish Heart Health Study found that moderate alcohol consumption was a small aid to heart health.

STUDY SUMMARY: The study was designed to measure the link between how much alcohol people reported drinking and coronary heart disease. This was a cross-sectional, random study of 10,359 men and women, ages 40–59, in 22 districts in Scotland. RESULTS: The rate of already-diagnosed coronary heart disease fell as the amount of reported alcohol ingestion increased. Among those with undiagnosed heart disease, there was a U-shaped result. (This means that the rate of heart disease fell with light-to-moderate drinking, then increased again with heavy drinking.) When the potentially protective effects of lifestyle, diet, and other factors were accounted for, the heart-protective benefits of alcohol diminished significantly. The researchers concluded that, "These results tend to confirm that intermediate alcohol consumption is a component of and contributor to a low coronary risk lifestyle."

CITATION: Woodward, M., Tunstall-Pedoe, H., "Alcohol Consumption, Diet, Coronary Risk Factors, and Prevalent Coronary Heart Disease in Men and Women in the Scottish Heart Health Study" *Journal of Epidemiology and Community Health* 49 (4): 354–62 (August 1995).

DOES ALCOHOL PROTECT WOMEN'S HEARTS AS WELL?

Medical researchers have been criticized, quite rightly, for focusing their studies on men. But males and females differ. Rather than being stuck with "hand me down" results from completely or predominantly male studies, women should be the subject of studies of their own. Researchers from the Centers for Disease Control and Prevention set out to see if alcohol was cardioprotective in females. Their results were published in the *Archives of Internal Medicine* in 1993.

STUDY SUMMARY: The study drew on the Epidemiologic Follow-Up Study of the First National Health And Nutrition Examination Survey (NHANES) to look at women ranging in age from 45–74. The women, who did not have heart disease when the study began, were followed for a mean of 13 years apiece. RESULTS: The women who reported drinking alcoholic beverages were 20 percent less likely to suffer from ischemic heart disease than were the nondrinkers. Even after other heart disease risk factors were accounted for, the drinkers did much better than the abstainers. The ones who drank between ½ and 2 drinks per day enjoyed the greatest benefits.

CITATION: Garg, R., et al., "Alcohol Consumption and Risk of Ischemic Heart Disease in Women" *Archives of Internal Medicine* 153 (10): 1211–16 (24 May 1993).

This earlier study, presented in the *New England Journal of Medicine* in 1988, had used women as test subjects for a look at alcohol's effects on heart health.

STUDY SUMMARY: For this study, 87,526 female nurses ranging in age from 34–59 were asked to report their consumption of alcohol on a dietary questionnaire. The women were followed until 1984, and the data were analyzed. RESULTS: The researchers found that drinking light-to-moderate amounts of alcohol offered protection against coronary heart disease. For example, the women who consumed 3–9 drinks per week had a relative risk of coronary disease of only 0.6 (or only 60 percent of the standard risk).

CITATION: Stampfer, M. J., et al., "A Prospective Study of Moderate Alcohol Consumption and the Risk of Coronary Disease and Stroke in Women" *New England Journal of Medicine* 319 (5): 267–73 (1988).

Although many researchers agree that alcohol, in moderate amounts, protects against heart disease, they have wondered who benefits the most. Everyone? Those who already have a low risk of heart disease? Or those with higher risks? A study appearing in the *New England Journal of Medicine* involving a large number of women found that most of the benefit went to those already at risk.

STUDY SUMMARY: This study, which began in 1980, involved 85,709 women ranging in age from 34–59. The women had not had heart attacks, angina pectoris, strokes, or cancer. They reported what they ate and drank, and were followed for 12 years. RESULTS: The light and moderate drinkers were less likely to die of cardiovascular disease. Heavy drinkers were more likely to die of breast cancer, cirrhosis of the liver, and other problems. The women most likely to benefit from light-to-moderate drinking were those who were either already at risk of heart disease or those over the age of 50.

CITATION: Fuchs, C. S., et al., "Alcohol Consumption and Mortality among Women" *New England Journal of Medicine* 332 (19): 1245–50 (1995).

The last study we'll look at wasn't specifically set up to look at the relationship between women's heart health and alcohol. Instead, it was designed to see how a variety of foods, including alcohol, influenced a woman's risk of heart disease.

STUDY SUMMARY: 287 women who had suffered heart attacks, ranging in age from 22–69, were involved. 649 controls who had serious diseases unrelated to ischemic heart disease were used for comparisons. RESULTS: There was a direct relationship between the risk of suffering a heart attack and the frequency of consuming meat, ham, salami, butter, coffee, and fat added to food. The risk dropped, however, with the consumption of fish, carrots, green vegetables, and fresh fruit. As for alcohol, moderate drinkers had a lessened risk of heart disease, while heavy drinkers had a greater risk.

CITATION: Gramenzi, A., et al., "Association between Certain Foods and Risk of Acute Myocardial Infarction in Women" *British Medical Journal* 300 (6727): 771–73 (1990).

ARE THE RESULTS VALID OR WERE WE FOOLED BY A STATISTICAL "TRICK"?

Although a considerable body of evidence suggested that alcohol was cardioprotective, and that light-to-moderate drinkers were actually better off than abstainers, some researchers felt that something was amiss. The data was skewed and the results misleading, they said, be cause many studies grouped abstainers and former drinkers together, then compared them to drinkers.

Grouping the abstainers and the quitters together was unfair, they felt, because many former drinkers had most likely been forced to quit after literally drinking themselves sick. Since the "sick quitters" were more likely to develop a variety of diseases and/or to die, mixing them with the nondrinkers polluted the "abstainers" category. It made the abstainers group look sicker than they really were—sicker than if the "abstainers" group had been limited to true, lifelong nondrinkers. Critics contended that if you accounted for the "sick quitters" who weighed down the "abstainers" group, the alleged benefits of drinking would disappear.

The "sick quitter" argument was addressed in a large-scale study appearing in the *American Journal of Cardiology* in 1986.

STUDY SUMMARY: Information was collected from 85,001 people between 1978 and 1982 in an attempt to answer key questions, including whether people who abstain from alcohol have a higher risk of coronary artery disease because they're grouped together with those who drank in the past. RESULTS: After controlling for the effects of age, sex, race, smoking habits, coffee consumption, and education, it was clear that former drinkers, those who drank very infrequently, and lifelong abstainers all had similar risks of developing coronary artery disease. In other words, the "sick quitters" were not weighing down the "abstainers" category with people who were already ill. These findings helped refute the idea that the "sick quitters" were inflating alcohol's cardioprotective abilities.

CITATION: Klatsky, A. L., Armstrong, M. A., Friedman, G. D., "Relations of Alcoholic Beverage Use to Subsequent Coronary Artery Disease Hospitalization" *American Journal of Cardiology* 58: 710–14 (1986).

The question was analyzed again and refuted by a 1991 study published in the prestigious medical journal *Lancet*.

STUDY SUMMARY: The relationship between coronary heart disease and alcohol consumption was examined in a study of 51,529 male professionals. The men filled out surveys regarding their medical history, heart disease risk factors, intake of food, dietary changes in the past 10 years, and alcohol consumption. Two years later, the men were again questioned about newly diagnosed coronary disease. RESULTS: Alcohol was found to provide protection against coronary disease, even when dietary fat and other heart disease risk factors were taken into consideration.

How about the "sick quitter" question? The researchers tested the data by removing all the current nondrinkers or those with disorders that may have led them to cut back on their alcohol consumption (the "sick quitters"). Still, the results remained substantially the same. In other words, "sick quitters" did not produce false results. Up to certain limits, alcohol does protect the heart.

CITATION: Rimm, E. B., et al., "Prospective Study of Alcohol Consumption and Risk of Coronary Heart Disease in Men" *Lancet* 338: 464–68 (1991).

Data taken from a massive study undertaken by the American Cancer Society provided further proof that "sick quitters" were not making it just appear as if alcohol protected the heart, and that moderate consumption of alcohol really did have a beneficial effect on the heart.

STUDY SUMMARY: The study began in 1959, when 276,802 men in the United States, ranging in age from 40–59, were enrolled. During the next 12 years 42,756 of the men died, 18,711 of them from coronary heart disease. The 55.3 percent of the men who were nondrinkers were used as references to develop age and smoking-stratified relative risks of dying of coronary heart disease. RESULTS: Nondrinkers were assigned a relative risk of dying of heart disease of 1.0. Occasional drinking produced a lesser risk of 0.86. The relative risk dropped as low as 0.74 among those who consumed 4 alcoholic beverages per day. The positive effects of alcohol remained, even when those who had been in poor health, or had a history of chronic disease, or who died during the first six years of the study were excluded. This shows that the positive effects of alcohol were not caused by including the "sick quitters" in the abstaining group.

CITATION: Boffetta, P., Garfinkel, L., "Alcohol Drinking and Mortality among Men Enrolled in an American Cancer Society Prospective Study" *Epidemiology* 1: 342–48 (1991).

Another 1991 study, this one appearing the *British Medical Journal,* addressed the "sick quitters" argument in a case-controlled study of New Zealanders.

STUDY SUMMARY: Two groups were involved in this study. The first included 227 men and 72 women who had survived heart attacks. They were matched against 525 men and 341 women serving as controls. The second group contained 124 men and 30 who had died of coronary artery disease, and a control group made up of 330 men and 214 women. RESULTS: Those who drank (up to 56 drinks per week) enjoyed a 40 percent drop in the risk of fatal and nonfatal coronary heart disease, compared with nondrinkers.

As for the "sick quitters" issue, those who gave up drinking had a lessened risk of non-fatal heart attacks compared to abstainers (but an equal risk of dying from coronary heart disease). These findings support the argument that consuming moderate amounts of alcohol reduces the risk of coronary artery disease, and refutes the notion that misclassifying "sick quitters" as abstainers has produced false results.

CITATION: Jackson, R., Scragg, R., Beaglehole, R., "Alcohol Consumption and Risk of Coronary Heart Disease" *British Medical Journal* 303: 211–16 (1991).

A 1993 study appearing in the *Journal of Public Health Medicine* addressed the same issue by examining data from the Oxford Vegetarian Study.

STUDY SUMMARY: The Oxford Vegetarian Study included some 6,000 people who did not eat meat, and about 5,000 who did. Since the participants had already answered questions about their drinking habits, and since the study included a "high proportion of lifelong teetotalers and ex-drinkers," researchers could use the data from the study to address the "sick quitters" issue. RESULTS: The authors were "unable to find a difference in the prevalence of risk factors between ex-drinkers and teetotalers . . ." The results of this study cast more doubt on the argument that alcohol only appears to protect the heart because "sick quitters" get mixed in the with healthy abstainers.

CITATION: Thorogood, M., et al., "Alcohol Intake and the U-Shaped Curve: Do Non-Drinkers Have a Higher Prevalence of Cardiovascular-Related Disease?" *Journal of Public Health Medicine* 15 (1): 61–68 (3 January 1993).

EXACTLY HOW DOES ALCOHOL PROTECT THE HEART?

It seems clear that light-to-moderate consumption of alcohol protects the heart, that it does so for both men and women, and that it is not a statistical quirk caused by "sick quitters." But how? How does ethyl alcohol, a substance that in large amounts is poisonous to the human body, protect the tireless pump that continuously circulates blood through the body?

A 1992 study published in the *Annals of Internal Medicine* found that alcohol exerted its beneficial effects by changing certain aspects of blood chemistry.

STUDY SUMMARY: 11,688 middle-aged men at high risk of coronary heart disease were studied. Several measurements were taken over a 7-year period to determine how much alcohol they each drank. The relative risk of dying from coronary heart disease was 1.0 in abstainers. In those who drank up to 7 drinks a week the relative risk dropped to 0.74; to 0.75 in those drinking up to 14 drinks a week; 0.5 in those consuming up to 21 per week; and 0.51 in those imbibing more than 21 per week. Statistical models applied to the data suggested that alcohol-induced increases in HDL were responsible for alcohol's ability to protect middle-aged men from coronary heart disease.

CITATION: Suh, I., et al., "HDL Cholesterol Contributes to Cardioprotective Effect of Alcohol" *Annals of Internal Medicine* 116 (11): 881–87 (1992).

HDL is the "good" cholesterol that helps to keep the arteries clear, allowing the blood to flow freely through the heart muscle and other parts of the body. We want the HDL to be high, so alcohol's ability to push it up is welcomed. In this 1992 paper published in *Circulation,* medical scientists "put a number" to alcohol's HDL-elevating properties:

STUDY SUMMARY: The researchers used certain models that analyze the various components of alcohol's protective effects while studying men in the Honolulu Heart Program. They concluded that about 50 percent of alcohol's beneficial effect is due to its ability to raise HDL. (They found that an additional 18 percent of the protection comes from alcohol's ability to lower LDL, the "bad" cholesterol that harms the heart, but this 18 percent protection was canceled out by an increase in systolic blood pressure caused by alcohol.) The researchers could not account for the other 50 percent of alcohol's helpful heart effects, speculating that it may be due to alcohol's ability to stop or slow the build-up of platelets, fibrin, and substances that can trigger heart attacks.

CITATION: Langer, R. D., et al., "Lipoproteins and Blood Pressure as Biological Pathways for Effect of Moderate Alcohol Consumption on Coronary Heart Disease." *Circulation* 85 (3): 910–5 (March 1992).

As the above study suggests, alcohol does do more than raise the HDL. The London Study also found that ethanol has other cardioprotective effects on the blood. It appears that alcohol's effects are not limited to increasing the "good" HDL. It also "thins" out the blood, thereby preventing unnecessary blood clots that could lodge in a coronary artery, abruptly cutting off the flow of blood and triggering a heart attack.

RESULTS: Researchers heading up the London (Northwick Park) Study found that alcohol consumption was inversely related to plasma fibrinogen concentration and platelet aggregability, and positively associated with plasma fibrinolytic activity. (These are measures of the blood's likelihood of clotting. While we want the blood to clot when we're bleeding, we want it to remain free-flowing and "thin" while in our arteries, lest a clot form and trigger a heart attack by damming up a coronary artery.)

CITATION: Miller, G. J., "Alcohol Consumption: Protection against Coronary Disease and Risks to Health." Proceedings on an International Symposium, "Alcohol and Cardiovascular Disease," Scheveningen, October 1991.

Not content to simply know that alcohol raises the HDL, researchers wondered how. What was the mechanism? And there's more than one "part" or "subfraction" to HDL: which of them was increased by alcohol ingestion? In a 1993 study published in the *New England Journal of Medicine,* researchers described what they had learned about the relationship between alcohol and the HDL.

STUDY SUMMARY: The study was designed to see if alcohol protected against coronary heart disease by altering the lipoproteins in the blood that are a part of the various cholesterol fractions. 340 men and women under the age of 76 who had had heart attacks were matched with an equal number of controls. None of the heart attack victims under study had a prior history of coronary disease, and all had been discharged from one of six Boston area hospitals. RESULTS: There was a significant inverse relationship between the risk of heart attack and alcohol consumption. In other words, as alcohol consumption rose (to a point), the risk of heart disease dropped. This was true even after accounting for other risk factors for coronary artery disease. Furthermore, alcohol consumption was associated with the levels of HDL, as well as the HDL-2 and HDL-3 subfractions. The authors concluded that alcohol's ability to increase the HDL-2 and HDL-3 subfractions plays a large role in protecting against heart disease.

CITATION: Gaziano, J. M., et al., "Moderate Alcohol Intake, Increased Levels of High-Density Lipoprotein and Its Subfractions, and Decreased Risk of Myocardial Infarction" *New England Journal of Medicine* 329 (25): 1829–34 (16 December 1993).

Finding a relationship between how much alcohol a group of people drink and their average HDLs is one thing; watching the HDL go up or down as volunteers increase or decrease their consumption is another. Scientists took this next step forward as they demonstrated alcohol's cardioprotective effects on the blood. This 1986 study, reported in the *British Journal of Nutrition,* clearly showed HDL going up as consumption of alcohol increased.

STUDY SUMMARY: This randomized, controlled, crossover study was designed to see how alcohol affected substances in the blood that played a role in ischemic heart disease. Some of the 100 subjects in the study drank alcohol (a mean of 18.4 grams per day) for 4 weeks, then drank no alcohol for 4 weeks. Others abstained for 4 weeks, then imbibed for the next 4. RESULTS: Alcohol was able to raise the protective HDL by up to 7, probably by pushing up the levels of HDL-subfractions (substances that "make up" the HDL). The researchers did not find an association between alcohol and plasma fibrinogen or other blood indices.

CITATION: Eastham, R. D., et al., "Alcohol and High-Density-Lipoprotein Cholesterol: A Randomized Controlled Trial" *British Journal of Nutrition* 56: 81–86 (1986).

This 1988 study published in *Lancet* confirmed that HDL rises and falls with changes in consumption.

STUDY SUMMARY: 12 healthy volunteers, all light drinkers, were enlisted to test the effect of alcohol on HDL and bile cholesterol saturation. During the study they consumed 39 grams of alcohol a day for 6 weeks, then abstained for another 6 weeks. RESULTS: Their HDL cholesterols rose significantly while they were drinking, then fell when they stopped. This study provided more proof that moderate alcohol consumption protects against heart disease by increasing the protective HDL in the blood.

CITATION: Thorton, J., et al., "Moderate Alcohol Intake Reduces Bile Cholesterol Saturation and Raises HDL Cholesterol" *Lancet* 819–22 (8 October 1988).

Although alcohol abuse is always dangerous and to be avoided, a group of men who drank to excess provided valuable information about alcohol and HDL. The study they participated in showed what happens to the HDL when alcohol is withdrawn.

STUDY SUMMARY: 26 men who abused alcohol, but were still healthy, were compared to controls matched for age and sex. When the 26 alcohol abusers entered into abstinence treatment, their protective HDL levels were high, which was good and was to be expected. But after two weeks of sobriety their HDLs fell back down to normal. The apolipoproteins AI and AII also fell from high levels at the beginning down to normal within two weeks. This study shows that alcohol influences several "parts" of HDL, and that abstaining can erase the alcohol-induced rise in the cardioprotective HDL.

CITATION: Kalbfleisch, J., et al., "Alcohol: High Density Lipoproteins, Apolipoproteins" *Alcoholism: Clinical and Experimental Research* 10 (2): 154–57 (1986).

What's Actually Happening inside the Arteries?

Most of the studies looking at alcohol and heart health present statistical probabilities: a given group of light-to-moderate drinkers has a lessened risk of heart disease, their HDL is higher than average, or their blood platelets are less "sticky." Group statistics are certainly interesting and encouraging, but what's actually happening inside the vital coronary arteries that supply fresh blood to the heart muscle? What happens when we move away from statistics and probabilities to actually examine the heart? This 1993 study presented in the *European Heart Journal* took a look, and found visual evidence of alcohol's protective effects on the heart.

STUDY SUMMARY: The coronary arteries of 484 men were studied by arteriography (the injection of dye into the arteries). The patients' artery disease was then rated according to the number of arteries with at least a 50 percent blockage. The amount of alcohol they consumed was determined by questionnaire. RESULTS: The "average coronary artery disease scores" went down as alcohol consumption went up. Even after age, smoking habits, and other variables were taken into account, alcohol had a protective effect on the coronary arteries.

CITATION: Ducimetiere, P., et al., "Arteriographically Documented Coronary Artery Disease and Alcohol Consumption in French Men" *European Heart Journal* 14 (6): 727–33, (1993).

Is It Really Alcohol, or Some Other Factor?

One of the great difficulties in scientific research involving human beings is dealing with a bewildering number of variables. It's easy to show, for example, that consuming alcohol pushes up the "good" HDL cholesterol. But other factors, such as exercise, can do the same thing. How do you know which deserves the credit?

One way to settle the issue is to use subjects who all have the same variable(s). In this case, researchers used a group of men who exercised. Since they all exercised regularly and vigorously enough to run a marathon, they could be used to settle the "alcohol or exercise" question. The lead author in this study, William Castelli, had served as director of the prestigious Framingham Study.

STUDY SUMMARY: The study involved 90 male physicians, all vigorous daily exercisers who participated in the 1979 Doctor's Marathon. They ranged in age from 27–68. The mean HDL-C level of the doctors was 55.6. The 14 who were nondrinkers had a mean HDL-C of 51.7; the 52 who consumed up to 6 ounces of alcohol per week had a mean HDL-C of 53.9; and the 24 who drank 6–18 ounces of alcohol per week had a mean HDL-C of 61.5. *Conclusion*: There was a clear relationship between the HDL-C and alcohol consumption—the greater the consumption, the higher the protective HDL-C. Since all of the doctors participating in the study were regular and heavy exercisers, this study showed that exercise alone was not raising the HDL.

CITATION: Castelli, W. P., et al., "Alcohol Consumption and High-Density Lipoprotein Cholesterol in Marathon Runners" *New England Journal of Medicine* 303 (20): 1159–61 (1980).

IS ONE TYPE OF ALCOHOLIC BEVERAGE HEALTHIER FOR THE HEART THAN OTHERS?

As early as 1904, physicians noted that drinking seemed to have a beneficial effect on the heart. In more recent years, the "French Paradox" has stirred up a great deal of interest. The French, who eat a relatively high-fat diet, have less heart disease than Americans. They also drink a lot of wine. People in some other countries drink a lot of beer or liquor, too, but do not seem to be enjoying the "French Paradox." Could it be that wine is the most powerful heart protector among alcoholic beverages? At first glance, that would seem to be true. The authors of a paper on this topic presented in the journal *Lancet* pointed to some factors that seemed to tilt the scales in favor of red wine:

REPORT SUMMARY: The authors of this paper reported that there may be other substances in wine, besides ethyl alcohol, that help protect the heart. They noted that red wine contains phenolic compounds with antioxidant properties. Experiments showed that phenolic substances in red wine significantly slowed the oxidation of human LDL. (LDL, the "bad" cholesterol that helps clog arteries, is more dangerous when oxidized.) In fact, the phenols from wine were better at inhibiting oxidation than was vitamin E, one of the major antioxidant vitamins.

This suggests that alcohol is only one of perhaps many cardioprotective substances in red wine.

CITATION: Frankel, E., et al., "Inhibition of Oxidation of Human Low-Density Lipoprotein by Phenolic Substances in Red Wine." *Lancet* 341 (8843): 454–57 (1993).

It's true that wine contains phenols and other substances that might conceivably make it a better heart protector than either beer or liquor. However, the weight of the scientific evidence to date suggests that *all* types of alcoholic beverages perform equally well when it comes to protecting against coronary heart disease. Here is one of the studies that found no significant difference between beer, wine, and alcohol. It appeared in a 1986 issue of the *American Journal of Cardiology*.

STUDY SUMMARY: Information was collected from 85,001 people between 1978 and 1982 in an attempt to answer key questions, including whether it mattered if one drank wine, beer, or spirits. The effects of age, sex, race, smoking habits, coffee consumption, and education were all accounted for. RESULTS: Beer, wine, and liquor all seemed to have equal heart-protecting abilities.

CITATION: Klatsky, A. L., Armstrong, M. A., Friedman, G. D., "Relations of Alcoholic Beverage Use to Subsequent Coronary Artery Disease Hospitalization" *American Journal of Cardiology* 58: 710–14 (1986).

The latest word available as this book is written comes from a review of the literature printed in the *British Medical Journal* on 23 March 1996. Researchers from Harvard, Kaiser Permanente, and the Erasmus University Medical School in the Netherlands reviewed 25 previously published studies on alcohol and the risk of coronary artery disease to see if one type of alcoholic beverage was better for the heart than another. They found that while some studies favored one type over another, "Most of the differences in findings . . . are probably due to differences in patterns of drinking specific types of alcoholic drinks and to differing associations with other risk factors. The study concluded that "The evidence suggests that all alcoholic drinks are linked with lower risk, so that much of the benefit is from alcohol rather than other components of each type of drink."

So it does not seem to matter whether you prefer wine, beer, or distilled liquor. They all contain ethyl alcohol, which appears to be the "active ingredient" responsible for protecting the heart.

DOES IT MATTER WHEN YOU DRINK?

It seems as if questions are never completely answered in medical research. That is, for each question answered, one, two, three, or more questions arise. When doctors noticed that people who drank alcoholic beverages seemed to suffer from less heart disease, they wondered if alcohol protected the heart. That question was answered "yes" in several studies. But this led to another puzzle: *How* did alcohol protect the heart? As researchers delved deeper into the subject, they discovered that, among other things, ethyl alcohol raised the beneficial HDL and HDL-subfractions ("components"). Answering the "how" question, naturally, led to yet another: When it comes to raising the HDL, does it matter when one drinks? Is sporadic heavy drinking as helpful as regular but light drinking? In other words, does downing a six-pack of beer every Saturday have the same effects as drinking one beer a day? The following study addressed that question:

STUDY SUMMARY: Researchers looked at 526 men who had coronary arteriography. The men were also categorized as "consistent" or "variable" drinkers. (For example, a consistent drinker might have a glass of wine with dinner every night, while a variable drinker may consume no alcohol for a week or two, then overdo it at a party.) RESULTS: Drinking alcohol was found to have an inverse, hence beneficial, relationship with coronary occlusion (blockages in the coronary arteries that supply fresh blood to the heart muscle). The lowest levels of coronary blockage were found among the regular and consistent drinkers. The abstainers, occasional drinkers, and variable drinkers had greater degrees of blockage. Not only that, but among the regular and consistent drinkers there was a clear relationship between the amount of alcohol consumed and the occlusion scores: Higher consumption led to less blockage. The variable drinkers, however, had higher occlusion scores no matter how much they drank. The results of this study show that consistent drinking will more likely protect the heart than inconsistent, variable consumption. In other words, slow and steady is better than binging.

CITATION: Gruchow, H. W., "Effects of Drinking Patterns on the Relationship between Alcohol and Coronary Occlusion" *Atherosclerosis* 43: 393–404 (1982).

RELATIVE RISK: ANOTHER WAY OF ASSESSING
THE BENEFITS

Relative risk provides another way of looking at the beneficial effects of moderate alcohol consumption on the heart. The relative risk is a complicated statistical model used in comparing the effects of an action. For our purposes, a relative risk of 1.0 means that you have the same chance of becoming ill or dying as do the people who drink a certain amount of alcohol (which varies from study to study). If the relative risk drops below 1.0, your odds of becoming ill or dying drop. The lower the relative risk, the better. As you will see in the studies that follow, the relative risk of suffering a heart attack drops as alcohol consumption increases.

You will also notice that no two studies have identical results. There are many valid reasons for the differences, including the following:

- the studies are designed differently
- some studies included only men, some only women, while others looked at both men and women
- different age groups were used
- some studies were adjusted for differences caused by age, cigarette smoking, and other factors; others were not
- there is a lack of standardization in the "alcohol consumed" categories, with some studies specifying the number of drinks, some noting the ounces of pure alcohol consumed, and others using "occasional," "light," or "heavy" drinker categories
- some studies treated all alcohol equally, others differentiated between wine, beer, and spirits
- various studies were conducted in different countries, where social and other factors may have affected the results

Don't be dismayed by minor differences in the results when looking at groups of studies. Instead, look for the general trends.

Alcohol and the Risk of Having a Heart Attack:
Case-Controlled Studies

These studies focus on the risk of having a heart attack and surviving. These are case-controlled studies, which means that the heart patients being studied were matched with a "control" group made up of people who were similar in many respects, but had not had heart attacks. (Using control groups for the sake of comparison makes a study more scientifically valid.)

Klatsky's 1974 study[1] looked at men and women in the United States, comparing those hospitalized for their first heart attack to other hospitalized patients. The study was adjusted to account for the effects of age, blood pressure, cholesterol levels, cigarette smoking, sex, and weight.

IF THEY CONSUMED:	THEIR RELATIVE RISK OF HEART DISEASE WAS:
less than 3 drinks per day	1.0
3–5 drinks per day	0.7
6 drinks per day	0.4

Statson's 1976 study[2] looked at men and women, ages 40–49, comparing those hospitalized for nonfatal heart attacks to other hospitalized patients. The study was adjusted to account for the effects of age, cigarette smoking, and sex.

IF THEY CONSUMED:	THEIR RELATIVE RISK OF HEART DISEASE WAS:
less than 6 drinks per day	1.0
6 or more drinks per day	0.6

Hennekens's 1978 study[3] looked at men, ages 30–70, comparing those who had died from coronary heart disease to people living in the community. The study was adjusted to account for the effects of cigarette smoking, religion, and weight.

IF THEY CONSUMED:	THEIR RELATIVE RISK OF HEART DISEASE WAS:
less than 3 drinks per day	1.0
3–5 drinks per day	0.7
6 drinks per day	0.4

Petitti's 1979 study[4] looked at women, ages 18–54, in the United States, comparing those who had had acute heart attacks to those of the same age who had not had heart attacks. The study was adjusted to account for the effects of elevated blood pressure, cigarette smoking, elevated cholesterol, gallbladder disease, and obesity. As you can see, drinkers had only about one third the risk compared to abstainers.

IF THEY CONSUMED:	THEIR RELATIVE RISK OF HEART DISEASE WAS:
(nondrinkers)	3.1
drinkers	1.0

Rosenberg's 1981 study[5] looked at women ages 30–49 in the United States, comparing those in the hospital for heart attacks versus other hospitalized patients. The study was adjusted to account for the effects of age, cigarette smoking, blood-fat levels, elevated blood pressure, the use or oral contraceptives, and obesity.

IF THEY CONSUMED:	THEIR RELATIVE RISK OF HEART DISEASE WAS:
(never drank)	1.0
currently drank	0.7

Ross's 1981 study[6] looked at women up to the age of 80, comparing those who had had fatal heart attacks to members of the community.

IF THEY CONSUMED:	THEIR RELATIVE RISK OF HEART DISEASE WAS:
(no alcohol at all)	1.0
less than 2 drinks per day	0.4

Siscovick's 1986 study[7] looked at men ages 25–75, comparing those who had suffered a heart attack to members of the community. The study was adjusted to account for elevated blood pressure, cigarette smoking, and activity levels.

IF THEY CONSUMED:	THEIR RELATIVE RISK OF HEART DISEASE WAS:
less than 1 drink per month	1.0
less than 1 drink per day	0.7
1–3 drinks per day	0.5

Kono's 1991 study[8] looked at men ages 40–69 in Japan, comparing those who had survived a heart attack to members of the community. The study was adjusted to account for the effects of age, blood pressure, exercise levels, diabetes, heart disease in parents, and job classification.

IF THEY CONSUMED:	THEIR RELATIVE RISK OF HEART DISEASE WAS:
less than 30 milliliters per day	1.11
30–59 milliliters per day	0.31
more than 60 milliliters per day	0.13

Those who never drank came out with a relative risk of 1.0 in this study, while former drinkers had only a 0.5 relative risk—half the odds as abstainers.

Jackson's 1991 study[9] looked at men and women ages 25–64 in New Zealand, comparing those who had suffered either nonfatal or fatal heart attacks to members of the community. The study was adjusted to account for the effects of age, elevated blood pressure, cigarette smoking, exercise habits, social class, and recent changes in drinking habits.

Among men ages 26–64 who had survived a heart attack:

IF THEY CONSUMED:	THEIR RELATIVE RISK OF HEART DISEASE WAS:
(no alcohol)	1.0
4 drinks or less per week	0.6
5–14 drinks per week	0.6

Among men ages 26–64 who died of heart disease:

IF THEY CONSUMED:	THEIR RELATIVE RISK OF HEART DISEASE WAS:
(no alcohol)	1.0
4 drinks or less per week	0.4
5–14 drinks per week	0.4

Among women ages 26–64 who had survived a heart attack:

IF THEY CONSUMED:	THEIR RELATIVE RISK OF HEART DISEASE WAS:
(no alcohol)	1.0
4 drinks or less per week	0.5
5–14 drinks per week	0.2

Among women ages 26–64 who died of heart disease:

IF THEY CONSUMED:	THEIR RELATIVE RISK OF HEART DISEASE WAS:
(no alcohol)	1.0
4 drinks or less per week	0.0–0.2
5–14 drinks per week	0.0–0.3

These and other case-controlled studies have somewhat different results, just as you would expect to see with any large group of studies. The overall pattern, however, is clear: the relative risk of suffering a nonfatal heart attack drops as alcohol consumption increases. *But remember: Heavy drinking is bad for the heart and terrible for overall health.* (And some of the heavy drinkers in this study whose hearts were healthy, courtesy of alcohol, undoubtedly suffered from other alcohol-induced ailments.) Moderation is the key. Small-to-moderate amounts of alcohol have potentially healthful effects on the heart, and can help to reduce the risk of heart disease in certain people.

Alcohol and the Risk of Having a Heart Attack: Cohort Studies

In addition to case-controlled studies in which "cases" have been carefully matched to "controls," medical and epidemiological researchers have also used "cohort studies" to gauge the effect of alcohol on the heart. Cohort studies typically follow large groups of people over many years. For example, 5,000 men and women may be enrolled in a cohort study. They would probably be divided into several groups depending upon how much alcohol they consume (none, 1 drink per day, 2 per day, et cetera). After a number of years, the researchers would tally the number of heart attacks in the "no drink" group, in the "1 per day" group, the "2 per day" group, and so on.

Like the case-controlled studies we've just reviewed, these cohort studies were published in prestigious journals such as the *New England Journal of Medicine,* the *American Heart Journal,* the *American Journal of Epidemiology,* and the *International Journal of Epidemiology.* And like the case-controlled studies, these cohort studies also suggest that moderate consumption of alcohol has a beneficial effect on the heart.

Yano's 6-year study[10] involved 7,705 men ranging in age from 45–66. The study was adjusted to account for the effects of age.

IF THEY CONSUMED:	THEIR RELATIVE RISK OF HEART DISEASE WAS:
(no alcohol)	1.00
1–6 milliliters per day	0.90
7–15 milliliters per day	0.67
16–39 milliliters per day	0.58
40 milliliters or more per day	0.46

Gordon's 22-year study,[11] published in 1983, involved 2,026 men ranging in age from 31–64. The study was adjusted to account for the effects of age, blood fats, weight, and the systolic blood pressure level.

IF THEY CONSUMED:	THEIR RELATIVE RISK OF HEART DISEASE WAS:
(no alcohol)	1.00
1–9 ounces per month	0.90
10–19 ounces per month	0.88
20–29 ounces per month	0.75
30–59 ounces per month	0.58
60 or more ounces per month	0.72

Gordon also examined 2,599 women, ranging in age from 31–64.

IF THEY CONSUMED:	THEIR RELATIVE RISK OF HEART DISEASE WAS:
(no alcohol)	1.00
1–9 ounces per month	1.05
10–19 ounces per month	0.68
20–29 ounces per month	0.72
30–59 ounces per month	0.75
60 or more ounces per month	0.76

Gordon's 1987 study[12] examined 1,910 men ranging in age from 38–55, following them for 18 years.

IF THEY CONSUMED:	THEIR RELATIVE RISK OF HEART DISEASE WAS:
(no alcohol)	1.00
1–9 ounces per month	0.63
10–19 ounces per month	0.68
20–29 ounces per month	0.67
30–59 ounces per month	0.62
60–89 ounces per month	1.00
90 ounces or more per month	1.40

Gordon also followed 823 men, ranging in age from 56–73, for 10 years. He found that:

IF THEY CONSUMED:	THEIR RELATIVE RISK OF HEART DISEASE WAS
(no alcohol)	1.00
1–9 ounces per month	1.10
10–19 ounces per month	0.93
20–29 ounces per month	0.77
30–59 ounces per month	1.00
60–89 ounces per month	0.74
90 ounces or more per month	0.62

Stampfer's 4 year study[13] involved 87,526 women ranging in age from 34–59. The study was adjusted to account for the effects of age.

IF THEY CONSUMED:	THEIR RELATIVE RISK OF HEART DISEASE WAS:
(no alcohol)	1.00
1–1.5 grams per day	0.7
1.5–14.9 grams per day	0.5
15–24.9 grams per day	0.6
25 grams or more per day	0.6

Miller's 7½ year study[14] involved 1,341 men in Trinidad, ranging from 35–69 years of age. The study was adjusted to account for the affects of age, systolic blood pressure, cholesterol levels, ethnic background, and smoking habits.

IF THEY CONSUMED:	THEIR RELATIVE RISK OF HEART DISEASE WAS:
(no alcohol)	1.0
1–4 drinks per week	0.83
5–14 drinks per week	0.46
15–59 drinks per week	0.31

Again, you'll notice that these cohort studies do not yield identical results. However, the overall trend is clear: Drinking moderate amounts of alcohol is associated with a lower risk of suffering a heart attack.

Alcohol Improves the Odds of Avoiding a Deadly Heart Attack

It seems clear that imbibing in moderation can help certain people to reduce the incidence of coronary heart disease. But what about heart disease mortality? Can drinking alcohol reduce the risk of *dying* of coronary heart disease? Several researchers have used cohort studies to look into this vital question. Here are some of the key findings.

The Chicago Western Electric Company Study,[15] which followed 1,832 men ranging in age from 40–55 for 17 years, was reported in the *Journal of Preventive Medicine* in 1980. The study was adjusted to account for the effects of age, diastolic blood pressure, cholesterol, heart rate, and smoking habits.

IF THEY CONSUMED:	THE RELATIVE RISK OF DYING OF HEART DISEASE WAS:
less than 1 drink per day	1.00
1 drink per day	0.95
2–3 drinks per day	0.90
4–5 drinks per day	0.67
6 or more drinks per day	1.83

Notice how the relative risk of dying of heart disease took a sudden turn up among the men drinking 6 or more drinks per day.

A 1981 study reported in the prestigious medical journal *Lancet*[16] followed 1,422 men, ranging in age from 40–64, in Great Britain. The study was adjusted to account for the effects of age, blood pressure, cholesterol levels, employment status, and smoking.

IF THEY CONSUMED:	THE RELATIVE RISK OF DYING OF HEART DISEASE WAS:
(no alcohol)	2.1
0.1–9.0 grams per day	1.0
9.1–34 grams per day	1.5
34 grams or more per day	0.9

A 1981 study reported in the *Annals of Internal Medicine*[17] followed 8,060 men for 10 years.

IF THEY CONSUMED:	THE RELATIVE RISK OF DYING OF HEART DISEASE WAS:
(no alcohol)	1.00
1–2 drinks per day	0.61
3–5 drinks per day	0.70
6 or more drinks per day	0.82

Notice that the best effect, that is, the lowest relative risk, was at 1–2 drinks per day.

A 1985 study reported in *American Heart Journal*[18] followed 1,184 men and women, ages 63 and up, for 4¾ years. The study was adjusted to account for the effects of age, cholesterol levels, sex, and smoking habits.

IF THEY CONSUMED:	THE RELATIVE RISK OF DYING OF HEART DISEASE WAS:
(no alcohol)	1.0
0.1–8.9 grams per day	0.3
9–34 grams per day	0.5
34 grams or more per day	0.8

Again, note that the relative risk drops with moderate drinking, but increases as the consumption goes up.

In Japan, Kono followed 5,477 male physicians for 19 years. He reported his findings in the *International Journal of Epidemiology*[19] in 1986. The study was adjusted to account for the effects of age and smoking habits.

IF THEY CONSUMED:	THE RELATIVE RISK OF DYING OF HEART DISEASE WAS:
(no alcohol)	1.0
an occasional drink	0.6
less than 54 milliliters	0.7
54 milliliters or more	0.7

A 1987 article in the *Journal of Chronic Disease*[20] reported on the results of a 15-year study involving 4,590 men and women, all over the age of 35, in the United States. The results for the men were:

IF THEY CONSUMED:	THE RELATIVE RISK OF DYING OF HEART DISEASE WAS:
(no alcohol)	1.3
1–30 drinks per month	1.0
31–60 drinks per month	1.3
61–90 drinks per month	1.5
91 or more drinks per month	1.5

Results for the women did not show as much variation:

IF THEY CONSUMED:	THE RELATIVE RISK OF DYING OF HEART DISEASE WAS:
(no alcohol)	1.1
1–30 drinks per month	1.0
31–60 drinks per month	1.0
61–90 drinks per month	1.0

An article titled "Alcohol Drinking and Mortality among Men Enrolled in an American Cancer Society Prospective Study" appeared in *Epidemiology* in 1990.[21] The article described the results of a 12-year study that followed 276,802 men, ranging in age from 40–59, in the United States. The study was adjusted to account for the effects of age and smoking.

IF THEY CONSUMED:	THE RELATIVE RISK OF DYING OF HEART DISEASE WAS:
(no alcohol)	1.0
an occasional drink	0.86
1 drink per day	0.79
2 drinks per day	0.80
3 drinks per day	0.83
4 drinks per day	0.74
5 drinks per day	0.85
6 or more drinks per day	0.92

The results of an 8-year study involving 123,840 men and women appeared in a 1990 issue of the *American Journal of Cardiology*.[22] The study was adjusted to account for the effects of age, education level, marital status, race, and smoking habits.

IF THEY CONSUMED:	THE RELATIVE RISK OF DYING OF HEART DISEASE WAS:
(no alcohol)	1.0
Less than 1 drink per month	0.9
Less than 1 drink per day	0.8
1–2 drinks per day	0.7
3–5 drinks per day	0.6
6 or more drinks per day	0.8

Finally, an article appearing in the British medical journal, *Lancet*[23], presented the results of a 2-year study that followed 51,529 American men, ranging in age from 40–75.

IF THEY CONSUMED:	THE RELATIVE RISK OF DYING OF HEART DISEASE WAS:
(no alcohol)	1.0
0.1–5.0 grams per day	0.99
5.1–10.0 grams per day	0.79
10.1–15.0 grams per day	0.68
15.1–30.0 grams per day	0.73
30.1–50.0 grams per day	0.57
more than 50 grams per day	0.41

The results of these and other studies strongly suggest that moderate amounts of alcohol lower the relative risk of dying of coronary heart disease. In other words, moderate imbibing may keep the heart beating longer.

THE J EFFECT

Most researchers agree that alcohol has a J effect on coronary artery disease. That is, if you plot the number of drinks people consume against their risk of developing heart disease, the result will look something like this:

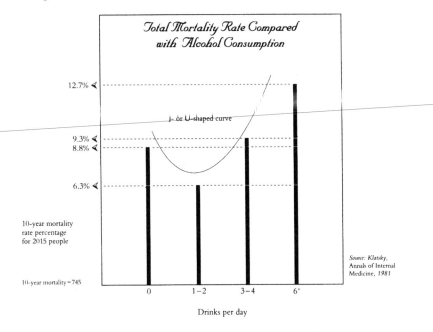

Total Mortality Rate Compared with Alcohol Consumption

J- or U-shaped curve

12.7%

9.3%
8.8%

6.3%

10-year mortality rate percentage for 2015 people

10-year mortality = 745

0   1–2   3–4   6⁺

Drinks per day

Source: Klatsky, Annals of Internal Medicine, *1981*

Nondrinkers have a relative risk of 1.0. The risk falls as the number of drinks increases and the J slopes down, then shoots back up as alcohol consumption increases beyond moderation.

Beware of the high end of the J! Heavy drinkers suffer from many problems, including an increased incidence of accidents, cancer, strokes, and death from all causes. The studies presented in this chapter only examined the relationship between alcohol and the heart, not alcohol and other diseases. And some studies have found either no benefit to the heart from drinking, or outright harm.

155

To Summarize the Scientific Evidence

The weight of scientific evidence supports the argument that light-to-moderate consumption of beer, wine, or liquor protects against coronary heart disease by increasing the protective HDL cholesterol and by "thinning" out the blood, thus making it less likely to clot unnecessarily. Alcohol also reduces stress and may lower the harmful LDL cholesterol. There may be other factors involved, including the antioxidants in wine, but more research is needed before we can definitively state that any of these factors play a major role in alcohol's protective effect against coronary artery disease.

Not all studies support the notion that alcohol guards against heart disease. That's to be expected, for different studies based on different designs using different methods, subjects, time scales, and means of analysis are bound to come up with different results. It is safe to say, however, that most medical scientists agree: Light-to-moderate consumption of alcohol can be good for the heart.

Appendix 2
Alcohol and Stroke
in the
Medical Literature

RESEARCHERS HAVE PUT numbers on the protective effects of alcohol, quantifying the potential benefits of light drinking as well as the risks of heavy drinking. The people or groups of people in these studies were assigned "relative risks" to represent the odds that they will have a stroke. The greater the relative risk, the greater the odds of suffering from or succumbing to a cerebrovascular accident. The lower the relative risk, the better. (Most studies assign a relative risk of "1.00" to nondrinkers or those who drink the least.) These studies were published in major scientific and medical journals, including the *American Journal of Epidemiology,* the *International Journal of Epidemiology,* the *American Journal of Cardiology,* and the *British Medical Journal.*

The studies looked at the risk of "total stroke," which included both blockage and rupture strokes, rather than the risk of either individual kind of stroke.

Klatsky's 1990 study,[1] published in the *American Journal of Cardiology,* followed 123,840 men and women for 5.3 years. The group had a mean age of 40.4. This study shows a J-shaped curve, with light-to-moderate drinkers enjoying a lessened risk of stroke as compared to abstainers and former drinkers. On the right or "high" side of the J, however, we see the heavy drinkers suffering an increased risk.

IF THEY CONSUMED:	THEIR RELATIVE RISK OF HAVING A STROKE WAS:
(nondrinkers)	1.0
(ex-drinkers)	1.0
less than 1 drink per month	0.8
less than 1 drink per day	0.8
1–2 drinks per day	0.8
3–5 drinks per day	0.7
6 or more drinks per day	1.4

Herman's 1983 study,[2] published in the *American Journal of Epidemiology,* looked at men and women ranging in age from 40–74. 132 cases hospitalized for their first strokes were compared to 239 control subjects. This study, which was adjusted to account for the effects of age and sex, shows that moderate drinking can slightly lower the risk of stroke.

IF THEY CONSUMED:	THEIR RELATIVE RISK OF HAVING A STROKE WAS:
(no alcohol)	1.0
less than 2 drinks per day	0.9
2 or more drinks per day	1.3

Cullen's 1982 study,[3] published in the *International Journal of Epidemiology,* followed 2,209 men and women over the age of 40 in Australia for 13 years. Again, the results show a small benefit for drinkers.

IF THEY WERE A:	THEIR RELATIVE RISK OF HAVING A STROKE WAS:
nondrinker	1.00
drinker	0.94

Paganini-Hill's 1988 study,[4] which was published in the *British Medical Journal,* followed 8,841 women, for over 17 years. The median age of the participants was 73. Again, mild drinkers enjoyed a small benefit.

IF THEY CONSUMED:	THEIR RELATIVE RISK OF HAVING A STROKE WAS:
(no alcohol)	1.00
1 drink per day or less	0.81
2 or more drinks per day	0.75

Gordon's 1987 study,[5] published in the *American Journal of Epidemiology,* followed 1,762 men ranging in age from 38–55 for 18 years. In this study, there was a sharp dip in the stroke risk for those consuming two drinks per day or less.

IF THEY CONSUMED:	THEIR RELATIVE RISK OF HAVING A STROKE WAS:
(no alcohol)	1.00
less than 2 drinks per day	0.29
2 or more drinks per day	0.92

Kozarevic's 1983 study,[6] published in the *International Journal of Epidemiology,* followed 11,121 men in Yugoslavia for 7 years. The men ranged in age from 35–62. This study shows that light-to-moderate drinking protects against stroke. And notice the difference between the last two categories: the ones who stop drinking *before* they become inebriated have a lower relative risk than do those who drink to drunkenness.

IF THEY CONSUMED:	THEIR RELATIVE RISK OF HAVING A STROKE WAS:
less than 1 drink per month	1.0
between 1 drink a month and 1 a week	0.4
more than 1 a week, up to 1 a day	0.3
1 or more a day, but not drinking to the point of inebriation	0.8
1 or more a day, drinking until inebriated	1.0

Stampfer's 1988 study,[7] published in the *New England Journal of Medicine,* followed 87,526 women in the United States for 4 years. The women ranged in age from 34–59. This study clearly illustrates the J curve, indicating that light-to-moderate consumption protects against strokes (but heavy drinking is dangerous).

IF THEY CONSUMED:	THEIR RELATIVE RISK OF HAVING A STROKE WAS:
(no alcohol)	1.0
less than 1.5 grams of alcohol per day	0.9
1.5–4.9 grams per day	0.6
5.0–14.9 grams per day	0.6
15.0–24.9 grams per day	0.5
25.0 grams per day or more	1.2

Klatsky's 1989 study,[8] published in *Stroke,* followed 10,751 men and women for an average of 3½ years. Seventy percent of the subjects were under the age of 50. This study looked at the risk of suffering blockage strokes (not total stroke or rupture stroke). The results pointed yet again to the protective effect of alcohol.

IF THEY CONSUMED:	THEIR RELATIVE RISK OF HAVING A STROKE WAS:
(no alcohol)	1.00
(former drinkers)	1.05
less than 1 drink per day	0.61
1–2 drinks per day	0.73
3 or more drinks per day	0.62

Klatsky's 1990 study,[9] published in the *American Journal of Cardiology,* followed 123,840 men and women, averaging 40½ years in age, for an average of 5.3 years. The stroke risk in this giant study fell as the amount of alcohol increased.

IF THEY CONSUMED:	THEIR RELATIVE RISK OF HAVING A STROKE WAS:
(no alcohol)	1.0
(former drinkers)	0.9
less than 1 drink per month	0.5
less than 1 drink per day	0.5
1–2 drinks per day	0.3
3 or more drinks per day	0.4

The studies did not come up with identical results, for each was different (they used subjects of different ages, sex, and health status; they had different measurements for the amount of alcohol consumed, et cetera). The overall pattern, however, is clear: Moderate amounts of alcohol offer a small but measurable amount of protection against stroke.

Notes

Chapter 1

1. Marian Burros. "In an About-Face, U.S. Says Alcohol Has Health Benefits," *New York Times,* 3 January 1996, A1.
2. Ibid.

Chapter 2

1. The distillers at Salerno weren't the first to distill ethyl alcohol out of alcoholic beverages: credit for that may belong to Indian distillers of the ninth century B.C., or the early Greeks. But the Salerno distillers were apparently the first to recognize its medicinal value.
2. Raimundo Lulio, quoted from *Alexis Lichine's New Encyclopedia of Wines & Spirits* (New York: Alfred A. Knopf, 1974), 6.
3. Hugh Johnson, *Vintage: The Story of Wine.* (New York: Simon and Schuster, 1989), 46.
4. The Gospel of St. Matthew, 26:27–29.
5. Hugh Johnson, *Vintage: The Story of Wine* (New York: Simon and Schuster, 1989), 81.
6. Ibid., 98.
7. Ibid., 477.
8. Ibid., 447–78.
9. Ibid., 396.
10. Joseph Kane, *Famous First Facts,* 4th ed. (New York: H. W. Wilson Co., 1981), 109.
11. Ibid., 109.
12. Ibid., 150.
13. *The Guinness Book of Records 1996 Edition* Peter Matthews, ed., Bantam Books, 1996. 478.
14. Ibid., 478.
15. Ibid., 397.

Chapter 3

1. Mario Frezza, et al., "High Blood Alcohol Levels in Women," *New England Journal of Medicine* 332 (2): 95–9 (1990).
2. *Macbeth,* 2.3. 32–33.
3. *Wines & Vines* 76 (7): 30 (July 1995).
4. Ibid., 18.
5. Ibid., 26.
6. Maurice E. Shils, James A. Olson, Moshe Shike, eds., *Modern Nutrition in Health and Disease Vol. II,* 8th ed. (Philadelphia: Lea & Febiger, 1994), 1081.
7. W. Rumpler, et al., "Ethanol and Dietary Fat Level Effects on Energy Expenditure in Humans," *Experimental Biology 95* (abstract), 1994.
8. C. Carmago, et al., "Alcohol Calorie Intake and Adiposity in Overweight Men," *Journal of the American College of Nutrition* 6 (1987): 271–78.
9. Loïe LeMarchand, et al., "Relationship of Alcohol Consumption to Diet: A Population-Based Study in Hawaii," *American Journal of Clinical Nutrition* 49 (1989): 567–72; Graham A. Colditz, et al., "Alcohol Intake in Relation to Diet and Obesity in Women and Men," *American Journal of Clinical Nutrition* 54 (1991): 49–55; C. Lieber, "Perspectives: Do Alcohol Calories Count?" *American Journal of Clinical Nutrition* 54 (1991): 976–82.
10. R. Klesges, et al., "Effects of Alcohol Intake on Resting Energy Expenditure in Young Women Social Drinkers," *American Journal of Clinical Nutrition* 59 (1994): 805–9.
11. D. F. Williamson, et al., "Alcohol and Body Weight in United States Adults," *American Journal of Public Health* 77: 1324–30 (1987).
12. See, for example, Graham A. Colditz, et al., "Alcohol Intake in Relation to Diet and Obesity in Men and Women," *American Journal of Clinical Nutrition* 54 (1991): 49–55.
13. Arthur L. Klatsky, et al., "Alcohol Consumption among White, Black and Oriental Men and Women," *American Journal of Epidemiology* 195 (No. 4): 311–23 (1977).
14. J. Istvan, et al., "The relationship Between Patterns of Alcohol Consumption and Body Weight," *International Journal of Epidemiology* 24 (3): 543–46 (1995).

Chapter 4

1. Katsuhiko Yano, Dwayne Reed, Daniel McGee, "Ten-Year Incidence of Coronary Heart Disease in the Honolulu Heart Program," *American Journal of Epidemiology* 119 (No. 5): 653–66 (May 1984).
2. Lawrence E. Ramsay, "Alcohol and Myocardial Infarction in Hypersensitive Men," *American Heart Journal* 98 (No. 3): 402–3 (1979).
3. Charles H. Hennekens, Bernard Rosner, Deborah S. Cole, "Daily Alcohol

Consumption and Fatal Coronary Heart Disease," *American Journal of Epidemiology* 107 (No. 3): 196–200 (1978).

4. Michael G. Marmot, M. J. Shipley, Geoffrey Rose, Briony J. Thomas, "Alcohol and Mortality: A U-Shaped Curve," *Lancet* 1: 580–83 (14 March 1981).

5. D. Kozarevic, N. Vojvadie, C. Kaelber, T. Gordon, D. McGee, W. Zukel, "Drinking Habits and Death: The Yugoslavian Cardiovascular Disease Study," *International Journal of Epidemiology* 12 (2): 145–50 (1983).

6. A. Dyer, J. Stamler, P. Berkson, M. Leper, H. McKean, R. Shekeele, H. Lindbert, D. Garside, "Alcohol Consumption, Cardiovascular Risk Factors and Mortality in Two Chicago Epidemiological Studies," *Circulation* 56 (1977): 1067–74.

7. Tavia Gordon, William B. Kannel, "Drinking Habits and Cardiovascular Disease: The Framingham Study," *American Heart Journal* 105 (No. 4): 667–73 (1983).

8. Paul White, quoted in *Health Issues Related to Alcohol Consumption*, P. M. Verschuren, exec, ed. (Washington, D.C.: ILSI Press, 1993), 83.

9. Richard D. Moore, Thomas A. Pearson, "Moderate Alcohol Consumption and Coronary Artery Disease: A Review," *Medicine* 65 (1985): 242–67; J. Veenstra, "Moderate Alcohol Use and Cardiovascular Disease," in Impacts on Nutrition and Health," A. P. Simopoulos, ed., *World Review of Nutrition and Dietetics* Karger, Basel, 65 (1991): 38–71.

10. Thomas Stuttaford, M. D., "The Benefits of Moderate Drinking," in *Drinking to Your Health: The Allegations and the Evidence*, D. Anderson ed. (London: The Social Affairs Unit, 1989), 34.

11. Erik Thaulow, Jan Erikssen, Leiv Sandvic, et al., "Blood Platelet Count and Function Are Related to Total Cardiovascular Death in Apparently Healthy Men," *Circulation* 84 (1991): 613–17.

12. N. A. Pikkar, M. Wedel, E. van der Beek, et al., "Effects of Moderate Alcohol Consumption on Platelet Aggregation, Fibrinolysis, and Blood Lipids," *Metabolism* 36 (1987): 538–47.

13. M. Seigneur, J. Bonnet, B. Dorian, et al., "Effect of the Consumption of Alcohol, White Wine and Red Wine on Platelet Function and Serum Lipids," *Journal of Applied Cardiology* 5 (1990): 215–22.

14. Michael G. Marmot, Eric Brunner, "Alcohol and Cardiovascular Disease: The Status of the U-Shaped Curve," *British Medical Journal* 303 (Vol. 6802): 565–68 (Sept. 7, 1991).

15. Eric B. Rimm, et al., "Prospective Study of Alcohol Consumption and Risk of Coronary Disease in Men," *Lancet* 338: 464–68. (August 24, 1991).

16. Katsuhiko Yano, George G. Rhoads, Abraham Kagan, "Coffee, Alcohol and Risk of Coronary Heart Disease in Japanese Men Living in Hawaii," *New England Journal of Medicine* 297 (No. 8): 405–9 (1977).

17. Arthur L. Klatsky, Mary Anne Armstrong, Gary D. Friedman, "Relations of Alcoholic Beverage Use to Subsequent Coronary Artery Disease Hospitalization," *American Journal of Cardiology* 58 (1986): 710–14.
18. Eric B. Rimm, R. Curtis Ellison, "Alcohol in the Mediterranean Diet," *American Journal of Clinical Nutrition* 61 (6 suppl.): 13785–825 (1995).
19. Eric B. Rimm, et al., "Review of Moderate Alcohol Consumption and Reduced Risk of Coronary Heart Disease: Is the Effect Due to Beer, Wine, or Spirits?" *British Medical Journal* 312 (No. 7033): 731–36 (23 March 1996).
20. P. M. Verschuren, exec. ed., *Health Issues Related to Alcohol Consumption* (Washington, D.C.: ILSI Press, 1993) 82.
21. Gary D. Friedman, Arthur L. Klatsky, "Is Alcohol Good for Your Health?" *New England Journal of Medicine* 329 (25): 1882 (1993).
22. "Alcohol" in the "Heart and Stroke Guide." American Heart Association, 1996.

Chapter 5

1. J. S. Gill, et al., "A Community Case-Control Study of Alcohol Consumption Intake," *International Journal of Epidemiology* 17 (3): 542–47 (1988).
2. Meir J. Stampfer, et al., "A Prospective Study of Moderate Alcohol Consumption and the Risk of Coronary Disease and Stroke in Women," *New England Journal of Medicine* 319 (5): 267–73 (1988).
3. J. Bogousslavsky et al., "Alcohol Consumption and Carotid Atherosclerosis in the Lausanne Stroke Registry," *Stroke* 21 (5): 715–20 (May 1990).
4. J. S. Gill, et al., "Alcohol Consumption—a Risk Factor for Hemorrhagic and Non-Hemorrhagic Stroke," *American Journal of Medicine* 90 (1991): 489–97.
5. H. Rodgers, et al., "Alcohol and Stroke—a Case-Controlled Study of Drinking Habits Past and Present," *Stroke* 24 (10): 1473–77 (January 1993).
6. H. Palomaeki, M. Kaste, "Regular Light-to-Moderate Intake of Alcohol and the Risk of Ischemic Stroke. Is There a Beneficial Effect?" *Stroke* 24 (12): 1828–32 (December 1993).
7. L. J. Berlin "Alcohol and Hypertension," *Clinical and Experimental Pharmacology and Physiology* 22 (3): 185–88 (1995).

Chapter 6

1. ACTH stands for adrenocorticotropic hormone.
2. Adrenalin is more formally known as epinephrine.
3. Jiang Wei, et al., "Mental Stress–Induced Myocardial Ischemia and Cardiac Events," *Journal of the American Medical Association* 275 (1996): 1651–56.

4. Thomas Stuffaford, M.D., "The Benefits of Moderate Drinking," in *Drinking to Your Health: The allegations and the Evidence*, D. Anderson ed. (London: The Social Affairs Unit, 1989), 34.
5. S. Renaud, et al., "Alcohol Drinking and Coronary Heart Disease," in *Health Issues Related to Alcohol Consumption*, P. M. Verschuren, exec. ed. (Washington, D.C.: ILSI Press, 1993) 84.
6. C. Baum-Baicker, "The Psychological Benefits of Moderate Alcohol Consumption: A Review of the Literature," *Drug and Alcohol Dependence* 15 (4): 305–22 (August, 1985).
7. P. H. Mansson, "Wine and Good Health," *Wine Spectator* 28 February 1989, 21–27.

Chapter 7

1. U. Keil, et al., "Alcohol Intake and Its Relation to Hypertension," in *Health Issues Related to Alcohol Consumption*, P. M. Verschuren, exec. ed. (Washington, D.C.: ILSI Press, 1993) 18.
2. V. Carins, U. Keil, et al., "Alcohol Consumption As a Risk Factor for High Blood Pressure: Munich Blood Pressure Study," *Hypertension* 6 (1984): 124–31.
3. U. Keil, T. Chambless, A. Hommerich, "Alcohol and Blood Pressure: Results from the Lubeck Blood Pressure Study," *Preventative Medicine* 18 (1989): 1–10.
4. Arthur L. Klatsky, et al., "Alcohol Consumption and Blood Pressure," *New England Journal of Medicine* 296 (No. 21): 1194–1200 (1977).
5. F. Facchini, et al., "Light-to-Moderate Alcohol Intake Is Associated with Enhanced Insulin Sensitivity," *Diabetes Care* 17: 115–119 (2 January 1994).
6. I. J. Perry, et al., "Prospective Study of Risk Factors for Development of Non-Insulin Dependent Diabetes in Middle Aged British Men," *British Medical Journal* 310 (6979): 560–64 (4 April 1995).
7. M. E. Weisse, et al., "Wine As a Digestive Aid: Comparative Antimicrobial Effects of Bismuth Salicylate and Red and White Wine," *British Medical Journal* 311 (7021): 1657–60 (1 January 1995).
8. J. Thorton, et al. "Moderate Alcohol Intake Reduces Bile Cholesterol Saturation and Raises HDL Cholesterol," *Lancet* 2: 819–22 (8 October 1996). See also these two studies: S. Kono, et al., "Prevalence of Gallstone Disease in Relation to Smoking, Alcohol Use, Obesity and Glucose Tolerance: A Study of Self-Defense Officials in Japan," *American Journal of Epidemiology* 136 (7): 787–79 (1992); Graham A. Colditz, "A Prospective Assessment of Moderate Alcohol Intake and Major Chronic Diseases," *Annals of Epidemiology* 1 (2): 167–77 (1990).
9. Sheldon Cohen, et al. "Smoking, Alcohol Consumption, and Susceptibility to the Common Cold," *American Journal of Public Health* 83 (No. 9) (Sept. 1993).

10. M. C. Dufour, et al., "Alcohol and the Elderly," *Clinics in Geriatric Medicine* 8 (1): 127–41 (February 1992).

11. P. A. Scherr, et al., "Light to Moderate Alcohol Consumption and Mortality in the Elderly," *Journal of the American Geriatric Society* 40 (7): 651–57 (1992).

12. "Patients Drink Beer in a Hospital Pub," *New England Journal of Medicine* 212 (11) (1935).

13. Matthew P. Longnecker, Brian MacMahon, "Associations Between Alcohol Beverages Consumption and Hospitalization, 1983 National Health Interview Survey," *American Journal of Public Health* 78 (2): 153–156 (1988).

14. A. Peruga, et al. "The Association Between Alcohol Consumption and Health Services Utilization," *Gaseta Sanitaria* 4 (18) 93–99 (1990).

15. T. Gordon, W. B. Kannel, "Drinking and Mortality. The Framingham Study," *American Journal of Epidemiology* 120 (1): 97–107 (1984).

16. Chart adapted from *Does Moderate Alcohol Consumption Prolong Life?* R. Curtis Ellison, M. D. (New York: American Council on Science and Health, 1993), 12–14.

17. Suminori Kono, Masato Ikeda, Shinkan Tokudome, Mashiro Nishizumi, Masanori Kuratsune, "Alcohol and Mortality: A Cohort Study of Male Japanese Physicians," *International Journal of Epidemiology* (Vol. 15, No. 4): 527–32 (1986).

18. A. G. Shaper, Goya Wannamethee, Mary Walker, "Alcohol and Mortality in British Men: Explaining the U-Shaped Curve," *Lancet* 2: 1267–73 (December 3, 1988).

19. Paolo Boffetta, Lawrence Garfinkel, "Alcohol Drinking and Mortality among Men Enrolled in an American Cancer Society Prospective Study," *Epidemiology* 1 (1990): 342–48.

20. Arthur L. Klatsky, Mary Anne Armstrong, Gary D. Friedman, "Risk of Cardiovascular Mortality in Alcohol Drinkers, Ex-Drinkers and Non-Drinkers," *American Journal of Cardiology* 66 (1990): 1237–42.

21. K. Cullen, "The Busselton Population Studies" in *Conference Proceedings, The Medicinal Virtues of Alcohol in Moderation* (Sydney, Australia 30 October–1 November 1991), 110–119.

22. Arthur L. Klatsky, Mary Anne Armstrong, Gary D. Friedman, "Alcohol and Mortality," *Annals of Internal Medicine* 117 (1992): 646–54.

23. R. Doll, "Alcohol and Health: An Overview" in *Conference Proceedings, The Medicinal Virtues of Alcohol in Moderation* (Sydney, Australia, 30 October–1 November 1991), 16–43.

24. L. O. de Labry, et al. "Alcohol Consumption and Mortality in an American Population: Recovering the U-Shaped Curve—Findings from the Normative Aging Study," *Journal of Studies on Alcohol* 53 (1): 25–32 (January 1992).

25. Mary Sunman, Sharon Hoerr, Homer Sprague, et al., "Lifestyle Variables

As Predictors of Survival in Former College Men," *Nutrition Research* 11 (2/3): 141–48 (1991).

26. Paolo Boffetta, Lawrence Garfinkel, "Alcohol Drinking and Mortality among Men Enrolled in an American Cancer Society Prospective Study," *Epidemiology* 1 (1990): 342–48.

27. Michael G. Marmot, M. J. Shipley, Geoffrey Rose, Briony J. Thomas, "Alcohol and Mortality: A U-Shaped Curve," *Lancet* 1: 580–83 (14 March 1981).

28. Arthur L. Klatsky, Mary Anne Armstrong, Gary D. Friedman, "Risk of Cardiovascular Mortality in Alcohol Drinkers, Ex-Drinkers and Non-Drinkers," *American Journal of Cardiology* 66 (1990): 1237–42.

Chapter 8

1. "Nutrition and Your Health: Dietary Guidelines For Americans," 4th ed., 1995. U.S. Department of Agriculture, U.S. Department of Health and Human Services, December 1995. Home and Garden Bulletin No. 232.

2. Marian Burros, "In an About-Face, U.S. Says Alcohol Has Health Ben efits," *New York Times*, 3 January 1996, A1.

3. USDA, HHS Release Updated Dietary Guidelines for Americans," Release No. 0004.96, 1.

Chapter 9

1. Hugh Johnson, *Vintage: The Story of Wine* (New York: Simon and Schuster, 1989), 103.

2. Gene Ford, *The Benefits of Moderate Drinking* (San Francisco, Calif.: Wine Appreciation Guild, 1988), 15.

3. Harold McGee, *On Food and Cooking. The Science and Lore of the Kitchen* (New York: MacMillan Publishing Company, 1984), 493–94.

4. Frank Bruno, Ph.D., *Psychological Symptoms* (New York: John Wiley & Sons, 1993), 8.

5. Paula Harris, "Cross Cultural Aspects of Drinking, Alcohol Abuse and Alcoholism" ASEV Online, http://www.winebiz.com/story2.html (24 June 1996).

6. Ibid.

Appendix 1

1. Arthur L. Klatsky, et al., "Alcohol Consumption Before Myocardial Infarction. Results from the Kaiser Permanente Epidemiological Study of Myocardial Infarction," *Annals of Internal Medicine* 81 (1974): 294–301.

2. William B. Statson, et al., "Alcohol Consumption and Non-Fatal Myocardial Infarction," *American Journal of Epidemiology* 104 (No.6): 603–8 (1976).
3. Charles H. Hennekens, et al., "Daily Alcohol Consumption and Fatal Coronary Heart Disease," *American Journal of Epidemiology* 107 (No.3): 196–200 (1978).
4. Diana B. Petitti, et al., "Risk of Vascular Disease in Women, Smoking, Oral Contraceptives, Noncontraceptive Estrogens, and Other Factors," *Journal of the American Medical Association* 242 (1979): 1150–54.
5. L. Rosenberg, et al., "Alcoholic Beverages and Myocardial Infarction in Young Women," *American Journal of Public Health* 71: 82–85 (1981).
6. Ronald K. Ross, et al., "Menopausal Estrogen Therapy and Protection from Death from Ischaemic Heart Disease," *Lancet* 1:858–61 (April 18, 1981).
7. David S. Siscovick, "Moderate Alcohol Consumption and Primary Cardiac Arrest," *American Journal of Epidemiology* 123 (No. 3): 499–503 (1986).
8. S. Kono, et al., "Alcohol Intake and Nonfatal Acute Myocardial Infarction in Japan," *American Journal of Cardiology* 68 (1991): 1011–14.
9. Rodney, Jackson, et al., "Alcohol Consumption and Risk of Coronary Heart Disease," *British Medical Journal* 303 (No. 6796): 211–16 (July 27, 1991).
10. Katsuhiko Yano, et al., "Coffee, Alcohol and Risk of Coronary Heart Disease among Japanese Men Living in Hawaii," *New England Journal of Medicine* 297 (No. 8): 405–9 (1977).
11. Tavia Gordon, William B. Kannel, "Drinking Habits and Cardiovascular Disease. The Framingham Study," *American Heart Journal* 105 (No. 4): 667–73 (1983).
12. T. Gordon, J. Doyle, "Drinking and Mortality," *American Journal of Epidemiology* 125: 263–70 (1987).
13. Meir J. Stampfer, et al., "A Prospective Study of Moderate Alcohol Consumption and the Risk of Coronary Disease and Stroke in Women," *New England Journal of Medicine* 319 (5): 267–73 (1988).
14. G. J. Miller, et al., "Alcohol Consumption: Protection Against Coronary Heart Disease and Risk of Health," *International Journal of Epidemiology* 19 (4): 923–30 (1990).
15. A. R. Dyer, et al., "Alcohol Consumption and 17-Year Mortality in the Chicago Western Electric Company Study," *Journal of Preventative Medicine* 9 (1980): 78–90.
16. Micheal G. Marmot, et al., "Alcohol and Mortality: a U-Shaped Curve," *Lancet* 1:580–83 (14 March 1981).
17. Arthur L. Klatsky, et al., "Alcohol and Mortality. A Ten-Year Kaiser Permanente Experience," *Annals of Internal Medicine* 96 (1981): 139–45.
18. Graham A. Colditz, et al., "Moderate Alcohol and Decreased Cardiovas-

cular Mortality in an Elderly Cohort," *American Heart Journal* 109 (No. 4): 886–89 (1985).
19. Suminori Kono, et al., "Alcohol and Mortality: A Cohort Study of Male Japanese Physicians," *International Journal of Epidemiology* 15 (No. 4): 527–31 (1986).
20. T. C. Camacho, et al., "Alcohol Consumption and Mortality in Alameda County," *Journal of Chronic Diseases* 40 (1987): 229–36.
21. Paolo Boffetta, Lawrence Garfinkel, "Alcohol Drinking and Mortality among Men Enrolled in an American Cancer Society Prospective Study," *Epidemiology* 1 (1991): 342–48.
22. Arthur L. Klatsky, et al. "Risk of Cardiovascular Mortality in Alcohol Drinkers, Ex-Drinkers and Non-Drinkers," *American Journal of Cardiology* 66 (1990): 1237–42.
23. Eric B. Rimm, et al., "Alcohol and Mortality," *Lancet* 338: 1073–74 (Oct. 26, 1991).

Appendix 2

1. Arthur L. Klatsky, Mary Anne Armstrong, Gary D. Friedman, "Risk of Cardiovascular Mortality in Alcohol Drinkers, Ex-Drinkers and Non-Drinkers," *American Journal of Cardiology* 66 (1990): 1237–42.
2. B. Herman, P. I. M. Schmitz, A. C. M. Leyten, et al., "Multivariate Logistic Analysis of Risk Factors for Stroke in Tilburg, The Netherlands," *American Journal of Epidemiology* 118 (No. 4): 514–25 (1983).
3. K. Cullen, N. S. Stenhouse, K. L. Wearne, "Alcohol and Mortality in the Busselton Study," *International Journal of Epidemiology* 11: 67–70 (1982).
4. Annlia Paganini-Hill, Ronald K. Ross, Brian E. Henderson, Postmenopausal Oestrogen Treatment and Stroke. A Prospective Study," *British Medical Journal* 297 (No. 6647): 519–22 (August 20, 1988).
5. T. Gordon, J. T. Doyle, "Drinking and Mortality. The Albany Study," *American Journal of Epidemiology* 125: 263–70 (1987).
6. D. J. Kozarevic, N. Vojvodic, T. Gordon, et al., "Drinking Habits and Death. The Yugoslavia Cardiovascular Disease Study," *International Journal of Epidemiology* 12: 124–50 (1983).
7. Meir J. Stampfer, Graham A. Colditz, Walter C. Willet, et al., "A Prospective Study of Moderate Alcohol Consumption and the Risk of Coronary Disease and Stroke in Women," *New England Journal of Medicine* 319 (5): 267–73 (1988).
8. Arthur L. Klatsky, Mary Anne Armstrong, Gary D. Friedman, "Alcohol Use and Subsequent Cerebrovascular Disease Hospitalizations," *Stroke* 20 (No. 6): 741–46 (June 1989).
9. Arthur L. Klatsky, Mary Anne Armstrong, Gary D. Friedman, "Risk of Cardiovascular Mortality in Alcohol Drinkers, Ex-Drinkers and Non-Drinkers," *American Journal of Cardiology* 66 (1990): 1237–42.

Bibliography

Books and Articles on the Health Benefits of Alcohol

Anderson, A. J., et al. "Pattern of Alcohol Intake and Blood Lipid Levels." *Alcoholism: Clinical and Experimental Research* 6 (1): 135 (1982).

Anderson, D., ed. *Drinking to Your Health. The Allegations and the Evidence.* London: The Social Affairs Unit, 1989.

Baghurst, K. I., Dwyer, T. "Alcohol Consumption and Blood Pressure in a Group of Young Australian Males." *Journal of Human Nutrition* 35 (4): 257–64 (1981).

Barrett-Connor, E., Suarez, L. "A Community Study of Alcohol and Other Factors Associated with the Distribution of High Density Lipoprotein Cholesterol in Older vs. Younger Men." *American Journal of Epidemiology* 115 (No. 6): 888–93 (1982).

Baum-Baicker, C. "The Psychological Benefits of Moderate Alcohol Consumption: A Review of the Literature." *Drug and Alcohol Dependence* 15 (4): 305–22 (August 1985).

Berlin, L. J. "Alcohol and Hypertension." *Clinical and Experimental Pharmacology and Physiology* 22 (3): 185–88 (1995).

Blackwelder, W. C., et al. "Alcohol and Mortality: The Honolulu Heart Study." *American Journal of Medicine* 68 (2): 164–69 (1980).

Boffetta, P., Garfinkel, L. "Alcohol Drinking and Mortality among Men Enrolled in an American Cancer Society Prospective Study." *Epidemiology* 1 (1991): 342–48.

Bogousslavsky, J., et al. "Alcohol Consumption and Carotid Atherosclerosis in the Lausanne Stroke Registry." *Stroke* 21 (5): 715–20 (May 1990).

Burros, Marian. "In an About-Face, U.S. Says Alcohol Has Health Benefits." *New York Times*, 3 January 1996, A1.

Carins, V., Keil, U., et al. "Alcohol Consumption as a Risk Factor for High Blood Pressure: Munich Blood Pressure Study." *Hypertension* 6 (1984): 124–31.

Camacho, T. C., et al. "Alcohol Consumption and Mortality in Almeda County." *Journal of Chronic Diseases* 40 (1987): 229–36.

Camargo, C. A., Williams, P. T., Vranizan, K. M., Albers, J. J., Wood, P. D. "The Effect of Moderate Alcohol Intake on Serum Apolipoproteins A-1 and A-II: A Controlled Study." *Journal of the American Medical Association* 253 (1985): 2854–57.

Castelli, W. P., et al. "Alcohol Consumption and High-Density Lipoprotein Cholesterol in Marathon Runners." *New England Journal of Medicine* 303 (20): 1159–61 (1980).

Coate, D. "Moderate Drinking and Coronary Heart Disease Mortality: Evidence from NHANES I and the NHANES I Follow-Up." *American Journal of Public Health* 83 (6): 888–90 (1993).

Cohen, S., et al. "Smoking, Alcohol Consumption, and Susceptibility to the Common Cold." *American Journal of Public Health* 83 (9): 1277–83 (1993).

Colditz, Graham A. "A Prospective Assessment of Moderate Alcohol Intake and Major Chronic Diseases." *Annals of Epidemiology* 1 (2): 167–77 (1990).

Colditz, Graham A., Branch, Laurence G., Lipnick, Robert J., et al. "Moderate Alcohol and Decreased Cardiovascular Mortality in an Elderly Cohort. *American Heart Journal* 109 (No. 4): 886–89 (1985).

Criqui, Michael H., Ringel, Brenda L. "Does Diet or Alcohol Explain the French Paradox?" *Lancet* 344 (8939-8940): 1719–23 (1994).

Cullen, K. "The Busselton Population Studies." In *Conference Proceedings, The Medicinal Virtues of Alcohol in Moderation.* Sydney, Australia, 30 October–1 November 1991.

Cullen, K., Stenhouse, N. S. Wearne, K. L. "Alcohol and Mortality in the Busselton Study." *International Journal of Epidemiology* 11 (No. 1): 67–70 (1982).

de Labry, L. O., et al. "Alcohol Consumption and Mortality in an American Population: Recovering the U-Shaped Curve—Findings from the Normative Aging Study." *Journal of Studies on Alcohol* 53 (1): 25–32 (January 1992).

Doll, R. "Alcohol and Health: An Overview." In *Conference Proceedings, The Medicinal Virtues of Alcohol in Moderation.* (Sydney, Australia, 30 October–1 November 1991), 16–43.

Doyle, J. T., Gordon, T. "Drinking and Coronary Heart Disease: The Albany Study." *American Heart Journal* 110 (2): 331–34 (1985).

Ducimetiere, P., et al. "Arteriographically Documented Coronary Artery Disease and Alcohol Consumption in French Men." *European Heart Journal* 14 (6): 727–33 (1993).

Dufour, M. C., et al. "Alcohol and the Elderly." *Clinics in Geriatric Medicine* 8 (1): 127–41 (February 1992).

Dyer, A. R., Stamler, J., Paul, O., et al. "Alcohol Consumption and 17-Year Mortality in the Chicago Western Electric Company Study." *Journal of Preventative Medicine* 9 (1980): 78–90.

———. "Alcohol Consumption, Cardiovascular Risk Factors, and Mortality in Two Chicago Epidemiologic Studies." *Circulation* 56 (1977): 1067–74.

Eastham, R. D., et al. "Alcohol and High-Density-Lipoprotein Cholesterol: A Randomized Controlled Trial." *British Journal of Nutrition* 56 (1986): 81–86.

Ellison, M. D., Curtis, R. *Does Moderate Alcohol Consumption Prolong Life?* New York: American Council on Science and Health, 1993.

Ernst, N., Fisher, M., Smith, W., et al. "The Association of Plasma High-Density Lipoprotein Cholesterol with Dietary Intake and Alcohol Consumption. The Lipid Research Clinics Program Prevalence Study." *Circulation* 62 (suppl. IV): 41–52 (1980).

Facchini, F., Chen, Y. D., Reaven, G. M. "Light-to-Moderate Alcohol Intake Is Associated with Enhanced Insulin Sensitivity." *Diabetes Care* 17 (2): 115–19 (2 January 1994).

Farchi, G., Fidanza, F., Mariotti, S., Menotti, A. "Alcohol and Mortality in the Italian Rural Cohorts of the Seven Countries Study." *International Journal of Epidemiology* 21 (No. 1): 74–82 (1992).

Folts, John D. "Spirits, Spice, Sticky Platelets and Heart Attack." The American Heart Association 21st Science Writers Forum, 1994.

Frankel, E., et al. "Inhibition of Oxidation of Human Low-Density Lipoprotein by Phenolic Substances in Red Wine." *Lancet* 341 (8843): 454–57 (1993).

Fraser, G. E., Anderson, J. T., Foster, N., Goldberg, R., Jacobs, D., Blackburn, H. "The Effect of Alcohol on Serum High Density Lipoprotein (HDL). A Controlled Experiment." *Atherosclerosis* 46 (1983): 275–86.

Frezza, M., Podava, C., Pozzato, G., et al. "High Blood Alcohol Levels in Women." *New England Journal of Medicine* 332 (2): 95–99 (1990).

Friedman, Gary D., Klatsky, Arthur L. "Is Alcohol Good for Your Health?" *New England Journal of Medicine* 329 (25): 1882 (1993).

Fuchs, C. S. et al. "Alcohol Consumption and Mortality Among Women." *New England Journal of Medicine* 332 (19): 1245–50 (1995).

Garg, R. et al. "Alcohol Consumption and Risk of Ischemic Heart Disease in Women." *Archives of Internal Medicine* 153 (10): 1211–16 (1993).

Gaziano, J. M., et al. "Moderate Alcohol Intake, Increased Levels of High-Density Lipoprotein and Its Subfractions, and Decreased Risk of Myocardial Infarction." *New England Journal of Medicine* 329 (25): 1829–34 (1993).

Gill, J. S., et al. "A Community Case-Control Study of Alcohol Consumption Intake." *International Journal of Epidemiology* 17 (3): 542–47 (1988).

———. "Alcohol Consumption—a Risk Factor for Haemorrhagic and Non-Haemorrhagic Stroke. *American Journal of Medicine* 90 (1991): 489–97.

Gordon, T., Doyle, J. T. "Drinking and Mortality. The Albany Study." *American Journal of Epidemiology* 125: 263–70 (1987).

Gordon, T., Kannel, W. B. "Drinking and Mortality. The Framingham Study." *American Journal of Epidemiology* 120 (1): 97–107 (1984).

————. "Drinking Habits and Cardiovascular Disease: The Framingham Study." *American Heart Journal* 105 (No. 4): 667–73 (1983).

Gramenzi, A., et al. "Association Between Certain Foods and Risk of Acute Myocardial Infarction in Women." *British Medical Journal* 300 (6727): 771–73 (March 24, 1990).

Gruchow, H. W. "Effects of Drinking Patterns on the Relationship Between Alcohol and Coronary Occlusion." *Atherosclerosis* 43 (1982): 393–404.

Harris, Paula. "Cross Cultural Aspects of Drinking, Alcohol Abuse and Alcoholism." ASEV Online, http://www.winebiz.com/story2.html, 24 June, 1996.

Heath, Dwight B., ed. *International Handbook on Alcohol and Culture*. Westport, Conn.: Greenwood Press, 1995.

Hennekens, Charles H., Rosner, Bernard, Cole, D. S. "Daily Alcohol Consumption and Fatal Coronary Heart Disease." *American Journal of Epidemiology* 107 (No. 3): 196–200 (1978).

Herman, B., Schmitz, P. I. M., Leyten, A. C. M., et al. "Multivariate Logistic Analysis of Risk Factors for Stroke in Tilburg, The Netherlands." *American Journal of Epidemiology* 118 (No. 4): 514–25 (1983).

Iliffe, S., et al. "Alcohol Consumption by Elderly people: A General Practice Survey." *Age and Aging* 20 (2): 120–23 (1991).

Jackson, Rodney, Scragg, Robert, Beaglehole, Robert. "Alcohol Consumption and Risk of Coronary Heart Disease." *British Medical Journal* 303: 211–16 (July 27,1991).

Kalbfleisch, J., et al. "Alcohol: High Density Lipoproteins, Apolipoproteins." *Alcoholism: Clinical and Experimental Research* 10 (2): 154–57 (1986).

Kaufman, D. W., Rosenberg, L., Hemrich, S. P., Shaprio, S. "Alcohol Beverages and Myocardial Infarction in Young Men." *American Journal of Epidemiology* 121: 548–54 (1985).

Kimball, Allyn W., Friedman, Lisa A. "Coronary Heart Disease Mortality and Alcohol Consumption in Framingham." *American Journal of Epidemiology* 124 (3): 481–89 (1986).

Klatsky, Arthur L., Armstrong, Mary Anne. "Alcohol Beverage Choice and Coronary Artery Disease: Do Red Wine Drinkers Fare Best?" *Circulation* 86: 34–42 (1992).

Klatsky, Arthur L., Armstrong, Mary Anne, Friedman, Gary D. "Alcohol Use and Subsequent Cerebrovascular Disease Hospitalizations." *Stroke* 20 (No. 6): 741–46 (June 1989).

————. "Relations of Alcoholic Beverage Use to Subsequent Coronary Artery Disease Hospitalization." *American Journal of Cardiology* 58 (1986): 710–14.

————. "Alcohol and Mortality." *Annals of Internal Medicine* 117 (1992): 646–54.

————. "Risk of Cardiovascular Mortality in Alcohol Drinkers, Ex-Drinkers and Non-Drinkers." *American Journal of Cardiology* 66 (1990): 1237–42.

Klatsky, Arthur L., et al. "Alcohol and Mortality. A Ten-Year Kaiser Permanente Experience." *Annals of Internal Medicine* 96 (1981): 139–45.

Klatsky, Arthur L., Friedman, Gary D., Siegelaub, A. B. "Alcohol Consumption Before Myocardial Infarction. Results from the Kaiser Permanente Epidemiologic Study of Myocardial Infarction." *Annals of Internal Medicine* 81 (1974): 294–301.

———. "Alcohol Use and Cardiovascular Disease: The Kaiser Permanente Experience." *Circulation* 64 (suppl. III): 32–41 (1981).

Klatsky, Arthur L., Friedman, Gary D., Siegelaub, A. B., Gerard, M. J. "Alcohol Consumption and Blood Pressure." *New England Journal of Medicine* 296 (No. 21): 1194–1200 (1977).

Kono Suminori, et al. "Prevalence of Gallstone Disease in Relation to Smoking, Alcohol Use, Obesity and Glucose Tolerance: A Study of Self-Defense Officials in Japan." *American Journal of Epidemiology* 136 (7): 787–79 (1992).

Kono, Suminori, Handa, K., Kawano, J., et al. "Alcohol Intake and Nonfatal Acute Myocardial Infarction in Japan." *American Journal of Cardiology* 68 (1991): 1011–14.

Kono, Suminori, Ikeda, Masato, Tokudome, Shinkan, Nishizumi, Mashiro, Kurotsuno, Masamori, "Alcohol and Mortality: A Cohort Study of Male Japanese Physicians." *International Journal of Epidemiology*: 527–32 (1986).

Kozarevic, D., et al. "Drinking Habits and Death: The Yugoslavian Cardiovascular Disease Study." *International Journal of Epidemiology* 12 (2): 145–50 (1983).

Langer, R. D. et al. "Lipoproteins and Blood Pressure As Biological Pathways for the Effect of Moderate Alcohol Consumption on Coronary Heart Disease." *Circulation* 85 (3): 910–15 (1992).

LaPorte, R. E., Cresanta, J. L., Kuller, L. H. "The Relationship of Alcohol Consumption to Atherosclerotic Heart Disease." *Preventative Medicine* 9 (1980): 22–40.

Lieber, C. S. "Metabolism and Metabolic Effect of Alcohol." *Medical Clinics of North America* 68 (1984): 3–31.

Longnecker, M. P., Berlin, J. A., Orza, M. et al. "A Meta-Analysis of Alcohol Consumption in Relation to Breast Cancer." *Journal of the American Medical Association* 260 (1988): 652–56.

Longnecker, M. P., MacMahon, B. "Associations Between Alcoholic Beverages Consumption and Hospitalisation, 1983 National Health Interview Survey." *American Journal of Public Health* 78 (2): 153–56 (1988).

Marmot, Michael G., Brunner, Eric. "Alcohol and Cardiovascular Disease: The Status of the U-Shaped Curve." *British Medical Journal* 303: 565–68 (1991).

Marmot, Michael G., Shipley M. J., Rose, G., Thomas, Briony J. "Alcohol and Mortality: A U-Shaped Curve." *Lancet* 1: 580–83 (14 March 1981).

Miller G. J., Beckles, G. L. A., Maude, G. H., Carson, D. C. "Alcohol Consumption: Protection Against Coronary Heart Disease and Risks to Health." *International Journal of Epidemiology* 19 (4): 923–30 (1990).

Moore, Richard D., Pearson, Thomas A. "Moderate Alcohol Consumption and Coronary Artery Disease." *Medicine* 65 (1985): 242–67.

Paganini-Hill, A., Ross, R. K., Henderson, B. E. "Postmenopausal Oestrogen Treatment and Stroke. A Prospective Study." *British Medical Journal* 297: 519–22 (1988).

Palomaeki, H., Kaste, M. "Regular Light-to-Moderate Intake of Alcohol and the Risk of Ischemic Stroke. Is There a Beneficial Effect?" *Stroke* 24 (12): 1828–32 (December 1993).

"Patients Drink Beer in a Hospital Pub." *New England Journal of Medicine* 212 (1935).

Perry, I. J., et al. "Prospective Study of Risk Factors for Development of Non-Insulin Dependent Diabetes in Middle Aged British Men." *British Medical Journal* 310 (6979): 560–64 (4 April 1995).

Peruga, A., et al. "The Association Between Alcohol Consumption and Health Services Utilization." *Gaseta Sanitaria* 4 (18): 93–99 (1990).

Petitti, D. B., Wingerd, J., Pellegrin, F., Ramcharan, S. "Risk of Vascular Disease in Women, Smoking, Oral Contraceptives, Noncontraceptive Estrogens, and Other Factors." *Journal of the American Medical Association* 242 (1979): 1150–54.

Phillips, N. R., Havel, R. F., Kane, J. P. "Serum Apolipoprotein A-1 Levels. Relationship to Lipoprotein Lipid Levels and Selected Demographic Variables." *American Journal of Epidemiology* 116 (No. 2): 302–13 (1982).

Pikkar, N. A., Wedel, M., van der Beek, E., et al. "Effects of Moderate Alcohol Consumption on Platelet Aggregation, Fibrinolysis, and Blood Lipids." *Metabolism* 36 (1987): 538–47.

Ramsay, L. E. "Alcohol and Myocardial Infarction in Hypersensitive Men." *American Heart Journal* 98 (No. 3): 402–3 (1979).

Renaud, S. C., Beswick, A. D., Fehily, A. M., Sharp, D. S., Elwood, P. C. "Alcohol and Platelet Aggregation: The Caerphilly Prospective Heart Disease Study." *American Journal of Clinical Nutrition* 55:1012–17 (1992).

Rimm, Eric B., Ellison, R. Curtis. "Alcohol in the Mediterranean Diet." *American Journal of Clinical Nutrition* 61 (6 suppl.): 1378S–82S (1995).

Rimm, Eric B., et al. "Alcohol and Mortality." *Lancet* 338: 1073–74 (Oct. 26, 1991).

Rimm, Eric B., Giovannucci, Edward L., Willett, Walter C., et al. "Prospective Study of Alcohol Consumption and Risk of Coronary Heart Disease in Men." *Lancet* 338: 464–68 (Aug. 24, 1991).

Rimm, Eric B., Klatsky, Arthur. L., Grobbee, Diederick, Stampfer, Meir J. "Review of Moderate Alcohol Consumption and Reduced Risk of Coronary Heart Disease: Is the Effect Due to Beer, Wine or Spirits?" *British Medical Journal* 312: 731–36 (1996).

Rodgers, H., et al. "Alcohol and Stroke—a Case-Controlled Study of Drinking Habits Past and Present." *Stroke* 24 (10): 1473–77 (January 1993).

Rosenberg, L., Slone, D., Shapiro, S., et al. "Alcoholic Beverages and Myocardial Infarction in Young Women." *American Journal of Public Health* 71: 82–85 (1981).

Ross, Ronald K., Mack, T. M., Paganini-Hill, A., et al. "Menopausal Estrogen Therapy and Protection from Death from Ischaemic Heart Disease." *Lancet* 1: 858–61 (April 18, 1981).

Rumpler, W., et al. "Ethanol and Dietary Fat Level Effects on Energy Expenditure in Humans." *Experimental Biology 95* (abstract), 1994.

Schatzkin, A., Carter, C. L., Green, S. B., et al. "Is Alcohol Consumption Related to Breast Cancer? Results from the Framingham Heart Study." *Journal of the National Cancer Institute* 81 (1989): 31–35.

Scherr, P. A., LaCroix, A. Z., Wallace, R. B., et al. "Light to Moderate Alcohol Consumption and Mortality in the Elderly." *Journal of the American Geriatric Society* 40 (7): 651–57 (1992).

Scragg, R., et al. "Alcohol and Exercise in Myocardial Infarction and Sudden Coronary Death in Men and Women." *American Journal of Epidemiology* 126 (1): 77–85 (1987).

Seigneur, M., Bonnet, J., Dorian, B., et al. "Effect of the Consumption of Alcohol, White Wine, and Red Wine on Platelet Function and Serum Lipids." *Journal of Applied Cardiology* 5 (1990): 215–22.

Shaper, A. G., Wannamethee, Goya, Walker, Mary. "Alcohol and Mortality in British Men: Explaining the U-Shaped Curve." *Lancet* 2: 1267–73 (1988).

Shaper, A. G. "Alcohol and Mortality: A Review of Prospective Studies." *British Journal of Addiction* 85 (Dec. 3, 1990): 837–47.

Shapiro, Laura. "To Your Health?" *Time Magazine,* 22 January 1996, 52–54.

Shils, Maurice E., Olson, James A., Shike, M., eds. *Modern Nutrition in Health and Disease Vol II*, 8th ed. Philadelphia: Lea & Febiger, 1994.

Siemann, E., Creasy, L. "Natural Compound in Wine Can Lower Cholesterol Levels." *American Journal of Enology and Viticulture* 43 (1992): 49–52.

Siscovick, David S. "Moderate Alcohol Consumption and Primary Cardiac Arrest." *American Journal of Epidemiology* 123 (No. 3): 499–503 (1986).

St. Leger, A. S., Cochrane, A. L., Moore, F. "Factors Associated with Cardiac Mortality in Developed Countries with Particular Reference to the Consumption of Wine." *Lancet* 1: 1017–20 (May 12, 1979).

Stampfer, Meir J., Colditz, Graham A., Willett, Walter C., et al. "A Prospective Study of Moderate Alcohol Consumption and the Risk of Coronary Disease and Stroke in Women." *New England Journal of Medicine* 319 (5): 267–73 (1988).

Statson, W. B., Neff, R. K., Miettinen, O. S., Jick, H. "Alcohol Consumption and Non-Fatal Myocardial Infarction." *American Journal of Epidemiology* 104 (No. 6): 603–8 (1976).

Suh, I., et al. "HDL Cholesterol Contributes to Cardioprotective Effect of Alcohol." *Annals of Internal Medicine* 116 (11): 881–87 (1992).

Suhonen, O., Aromas, A., Reunanen, A., Knekt, P. "Alcohol Consumption and Sudden Coronary Death in Middle-Aged Finnish Men." *Acta Medica Scandinavia* 221 (1987): 335–41.

Sunman, Mary, Hoerr, Sharon, Sprague, Homer, et al. "Lifestyle Variables As Predictors of Survival in Former College Men." *Nutrition Research* 11 (2/3): 141–48 (1991).

Thaulow, E., Erikssen, J., Sandvic, L., et al. "Blood Platelet Count and Function Are Related to Total Cardiovascular Death in Apparently Healthy Men." *Circulation* 84 (1991): 613–17.

Thorogood, M., et al. "Alcohol Intake and the U-Shaped Curve: Do Non-Drinkers Have a Higher Prevalence of Cardiovascular-Related Disease?" *Journal of Public Health Medicine* 15 (1): 61–68 (1993).

Thorton, J., et al. "Moderate Alcohol Intake Reduces Bile Cholesterol Saturation and Raises HDL Cholesterol." *Lancet* ii: 819–22 (8 October 1986).

Turner, T. B., et al. "The Beneficial Side of Moderate Alcohol Use." *Johns Hopkins Medical Journal* 148 (2): 53–63 (1981).

Valimaki, M., Nikkila, E. A., Taskinen, M. R., Tlikarhi, R. "Rapid Decrease in High Density Lipoprotein Subfraction and Postheparin Plasma Lipase Activities after Cessation of Chronic Alcohol Intake." *Atherosclerosis* 59 (1986): 147–53.

Vasisht, S., et al. "Effect of Alcohol on Serum Lipids and Lipoproteins in Male Drinkers." *Indian Journal of Medical Research* 96 (1992): 333–37.

Veenstra, J. "Moderate Alcohol Use and Coronary Heart Disease; a U-Shaped Curve?" in Simopoulos, A. P., ed. "Impacts on Nutrition and Health." *World Review of Nutrition and Dietetics* Karger, Basel, 65 (1991): 38–39.

Verschuren, P. M., exec. ed. *Health Issues Related to Alcohol Consumption.* Washington, D.C.: ILSI Press, 1993.

Voelker, R. "Nocebos Contribute to a Host of Ills." *Journal of the American Medical Association* 275 (5)(1966).

Wei J., et al. "Mental Stress-Induced Myocardial Ischemia and Cardiac Events." *Journal of the American Medical Association* 275 (1996): 1651–56.

Weisse, M. E., et al. "Wine As a Digestive Aid: Comparative Antimicrobial Effects of Bismuth Salicylate and Red and White Wine." *British Medical Journal* 311 (7021): 1657–60 (1 January 1995).

Willett, Walter, Hennekens, Charles H., Siegel, A. J., Adner, M. M., Castelli, W. P. "Alcohol Consumption and High Density Lipoprotein Cholesterol in Marathon Runners." *New England Journal of Medicine* 303: 1159–61 (1980).

Willett, Walter, Stampfer, Meir J., Colditz, Graham A., Rosner, Bernard, Hennekens, Charles H., Speizer, Frank E. "Moderate Alcohol Consumption and Risk of Breast Cancer." *New England Journal of Medicine* 316 (No. 19): 1174–80 (1987).

Woodward, M., Tunstall-Pedoe, H. "Alcohol Consumption, Diet, Coronary Risk Factors, and Prevalent Coronary Heart Disease in Men and Women in the Scottish Heart Health Study." *Journal of Epidemioloy and Community Health* 49 (4): 354–62 (1995).

Yano, Katsuhiko, Rhoads, George G., Kagan, Abraham. "Coffee, Alcohol and Risk of Coronary Heart Disease among Japanese Men Living in Hawaii." *New England Journal of Medicine* 297 (No. 8): 405–9 (1977).

Yano, Katsuhiko, Reed, Dwayne, McGee, Daniel "Ten-Year Incidence of Coronary Heart Disease in the Honolulu Heart Program." *American Journal of Epidemiology* 119 (No. 5): 653–66 (May 1984).

Eating for Health

Carper, Jean. *The Food Pharmacy*. New York: Bantam Books, 1988.

Fox, Arnold. *The Beverly Hills Medical Diet*. New York: Bantam Books, 1982.

Fox, Arnold, and Fox, Barry. *Beyond Positive Thinking*. Carson, Calif.: Hay House, 1991.

———. *Immune For Life*. Rocklin, Calif.: Prima Publishing and Communications, 1989.

———. *Making Miracles*. Random Ho Hindah Press, 1995.

———. *Wake Up! You're Alive*. Deerfield Beach, Fla: Health Communications, 1989.

Fox, Barry. *Foods to Heal By*. New York: St. Martin's Press, 1997.

Mindell, Earl. *Food As Medicine*. New York: Fireside Books, 1994.

Murray, Michael. *The Healing Power of Foods*. Rocklin, Calif.: Prima Publishing and Communications, 1993.

Selye, Hans. *Stress Without Distress*. New York: New American Library, 1974.

Werback, Melvyn, ed. *Nutritional Influences on Illness*. 2nd Edition. Tarzana, Calif.: Third Line Press, 1993.

Woteki, Catherine, and Thomas, Paul, eds. *Eat for Life. The Food and Nutrition Board's Guide to Reducing Your Risk of Chronic Disease*. Washington, D.C.: National Academy Press, 1992.